THE TRUTH ABOUT
EATING DISORDERS

THE TRUTH ABOUT EATING DISORDERS

SECOND EDITION

ROBERT N. GOLDEN, M.D.
University of Wisconsin–Madison
General Editor

FRED L. PETERSON, PH.D.
University of Texas–Austin
General Editor

GERRI FREID KRAMER
Principal Author

WILLIAM KANE, PH.D.
University of New Mexico
Adviser to the First Edition

MARK J. KITTLESON, PH.D.
Southern Illinois University
Adviser to the First Edition

Facts On File
An imprint of Infobase Publishing

The Truth About Eating Disorders, Second Edition

Facts On File, Inc.
An imprint of Infobase Publishing
132 West 31st Street
New York NY 10001

Library of Congress Cataloging-in-Publication Data

The truth about eating disorders / Robert N. Golden, general editor; Frank L. Peterson, general editor; Gerri Freid Kramer, principal author.—2nd ed.
p. cm.
Includes bibliographical references and index.
ISBN-13: 978-0-8160-7633-8 (hardcover: alk. paper)
ISBN-10: 0-8160-7633-2 (hardcover: alk. paper)   1. Eating disorders—Popular works.
I. Kramer, Gerri Freid.

RC552.E18T78 2009
616.85′26—dc22

2008044036

Facts On File books are available at special discounts when purchased in bulk quantities for businesses, associations, institutions or sales promotions. Please call our Special Sales Department in New York at (212) 967-8800 or (800) 322-8755.

You can find Facts On File on the World Wide Web at
http://www.factsonfile.com

Text design by David Strelecky

Printed and bound in United States of America

MP KC 10 9 8 7 6 5 4 3 2 1

This book is printed on acid-free paper and contains 30 percent postconsumer content.

CONTENTS

List of Illustrations   vii

Preface   ix

How to Use This Book   xiii

Normal Behaviors and Eating Disorders   1

A to Z Entries   **13**

   Anorexia   15

   Bigorexia/Muscle Dysmorphia   21

   Binge-Eating Disorder   25

   Bulimia   31

   Caloric Intake and Expenditures   38

   Depression and Weight   42

   Diet Pills   49

   Eating Disorders, Causes of   54

   Eating Disorders, Symptoms and Diagnosis of   62

   Eating Disorders in Men and Boys   71

   Ethnicity, Genetics, and Eating Disorders   75

   Exercise   83

   Fad Diets   90

   Food Allergies   98

Internet and Eating Disorders, The   103
Laxative Abuse   108
Media and Eating Disorders   112
Morbidity and Mortality   121
Nutrition and Nutritional Deficiencies   125
Obesity   135
Peer Pressure   145
Purging   149
Self-Image   153
Stress and Eating Habits   158
Treatment   163
Weight Control   174
Women and Eating Disorders   177

Hotlines and Help Sites   183
Glossary   189
Index   199

LIST OF ILLUSTRATIONS

Students Who Have Used Anabolic Steroids
at Least Once in Their Lifetime   25

How High School Students Tried to Lose
or Avoid Gaining Weight   33

High School Students and Depression   44

Comparing the Average Model
to the Average American Woman   59

High School Student Participation in Physical Activity   85

Where Americans Get Nutrition Information   96

Comparing American Females to Their TV Counterparts   113

How Many Young People Are Overweight or At Risk?   126

How High School Students Eat   128

The Food Guide Pyramids   131–132

BMI Distribution Among Adults Aged 20–74 Years:
1980 and 2006   138

The Body Mass Index   139

Students Trying to Lose Weight   142

The Effectiveness of Treatment for Eating Disorders   171

PREFACE

The Truth About series—updated and expanded to include 20 volumes—seeks to identify the most pressing health issues and social challenges confronting our nation's youth. Adolescence is the period between the onset of puberty and the attainment of adulthood. Adolescence is also a time of storm, stress, and risk-taking for many young people. During adolescence, a person's health is influenced by biological, psychological, and social factors, all of which interact with one's environment—family, peers, school, and community. It is a time when teenagers experience profound changes.

With the latest available statistics and new insights that have emerged from ongoing research, the Truth About series seeks to help young people build a foundation of information as they face some of the challenges that will affect their health and well-being. These challenges include high-risk behaviors, such as drinking, smoking, and other drug use; sexual behaviors that can lead to adolescent pregnancy and sexually transmitted diseases (STDs), such as HIV/AIDS; mental health concerns, such as depression and suicide; learning disorders and disabilities, which are often associated with school failures and school dropouts; serious family problems, including domestic violence and abuse; and lifestyle factors, which increase adolescents' risk for noncommunicable diseases, such as diabetes and cardiovascular disease, among others.

Broader underlying factors also influence adolescent health. These include socioeconomic circumstances, such as poverty, available health care, and the political and social situations in which young people live. Although these factors can negatively affect adolescent health and well-being, as well as school performance, many of these negative health outcomes are preventable with the proper knowledge and information.

With prevention in mind, the writers and editors of each topical volume in the Truth About series have tried to provide cutting-edge information that is supported by research and scientific evidence. Vital facts are presented that inform youth about the challenges experienced during adolescence, while special features seek to dispel common myths and misconceptions. Some of the main topics explored include abuse, alcohol, death and dying, divorce, drugs, eating disorders, family life, fear and depression, rape, sexual behavior and unplanned pregnancy, smoking, and violence. All volumes discuss risk-taking behaviors and their consequences, healthy choices, prevention, available treatments, and where to get help.

In this new edition of the series, we also have added eight new titles in areas of increasing significance to today's youth. ADHD, or attention-deficit/hyperactivity disorder, and other learning disorders are diagnosed with increasing frequency, and many students have observed or know of classmates receiving treatment for these conditions, even if they have not themselves received this diagnosis. Gambling is gaining currency in our culture, as casinos open and expand in many parts of the country, and the Internet offers easy access for this addictive behavior. Another consequence of our increasingly "online" society, unfortunately, is the presence of online predators. Environmental hazards represent yet another danger, and it is important to provide unbiased information about this topic to our youth. Suicide, which for many years has been a "silent epidemic," is now gaining recognition as a major public health problem throughout the life span, including the teenage and young adult years. We now also offer an overview of illness and disease in a volume that includes the major conditions of particular interest and concern to youth. In addition to illness, however, it is essential to emphasize health and its promotion, and this is especially apparent in the volumes on physical fitness and stress management.

It is our intent that each book serve as an accessible, authoritative resource that young people can turn to for accurate and meaningful answers to their specific questions. The series can help them research particular problems and provide an up-to-date evidence base. It is also designed with parents, teachers, and counselors in mind so that they have a reliable resource that they can share with youth who seek their guidance.

Finally, we have tried to provide unbiased facts rather than subjective opinions. Our goal is to help elevate the health of the public with an emphasis on its most precious component—our youth. As young people face the challenges of an increasingly complex world, we as educators want them to be armed with the most powerful weapon available—knowledge.

Robert N. Golden, M.D.
Fred L. Peterson, Ph.D.
General Editors

HOW TO USE THIS BOOK

NOTE TO STUDENTS

Knowledge is power. By possessing knowledge you have the ability to make decisions, ask follow-up questions, or know where to go to obtain more information. In the world of health that is power! That is the purpose of this book—to provide you the power you need to obtain unbiased, accurate information and *The Truth About Eating Disorders*.

Topics in each volume of The Truth About are arranged in alphabetical order, from A to Z. Each of these entries defines its topic and explains in detail the particular issue. At the end of most entries are cross-references to related topics. A list of all topics by letter can be found in the table of contents or at the back of the book in the index.

How have these books been compiled? First, the publisher worked with me to identify some of the country's leading authorities on key issues in health education. These individuals were asked to identify some of the major concerns that young people have about such topics. The writers read the literature, spoke with health experts, and incorporated their own life and professional experiences to pull together the most up-to-date information on health issues, particularly those of interest to adolescents and of concern in *Healthy People 2010*.

Throughout the alphabetical entries, the reader will find sidebars that separate fact from fiction. There are question-and-answer boxes that attempt to address the most common questions that youth ask about sensitive topics. In addition, readers will find a special feature called "Teens Speak"—case studies of teens with personal stories related to the topic in hand.

This may be one of the most important books you will ever read. Please share it with your friends, families, teachers, and classmates. Remember, you possess the power to control your future. One way to affect your course is through the acquisition of knowledge. Good luck and keep healthy.

NOTE TO LIBRARIANS

This book, along with the rest of the series, The Truth About, serves as a wonderful resource for young researchers. It contains a variety of facts, case studies, and further readings that the reader can use to help answer questions, formulate new questions, or determine where to go to find more information. Even though the topics may be considered delicate by some, do not be afraid to ask patrons if they have questions. Feel free to direct them to the appropriate sources, but do not press them if you encounter reluctance. The best we can do as educators is to let young people know that we are there when they need us.

Mark J. Kittleson, Ph.D.
Adviser to the First Edition

NORMAL BEHAVIORS AND EATING DISORDERS

Have you ever eaten when you weren't hungry, just because something tasted really good? Have you ever been too nervous or too upset to eat anything at all? Have you found yourself back at the refrigerator for a third time while struggling through a research paper? Maybe you've compared yourself to your friends and your family members and wondered whether your eating habits were normal. Statistically speaking, your eating habits are probably perfectly normal. Feelings and emotions often affect how often and how much people eat.

When you're in your teens, or at any other age, really, it's normal to think about food often—just as it's normal *not* to think about food very often. How large a role food plays in your life will vary based on your upbringing, your personality, and your likes and dislikes. Sometimes, though, food becomes a true obsession, and the result is an eating disorder. Eating disorders are serious illnesses that usually involve eating way too little or way too much, and they can seriously endanger one's health.

At one time, eating disorders were rarely mentioned and poorly understood. Today experts throughout the world openly research, treat, and discuss eating disorders. These efforts have challenged many early assumptions about eating disorders. For example, the idea that they are limited to young, white girls has been debunked. Although many young, white girls suffer from eating disorders, they affect people regardless of gender, ethnicity, and age.

Experts now know that eating disorders are mental health diseases that have recognizable causes, clear symptoms, and predictable outcomes. They also respond to treatment.

Because experts believe many cases go unreported, it is difficult to accurately quantify exactly how many Americans suffer from eating disorders. The National Association of Anorexia Nervosa and Associated Eating Disorders (ANAD) reports that the incidence of eating disorders in the United States has reached "epidemic levels," namely 7 million women and 1 million men. The National Eating Disorders Association (NEDA) puts the estimate even higher, reporting that 10 million women and 1 million men suffer from anorexia and bulimia and that millions more have binge-eating disorder. All estimates show that the great majority of sufferers are female, but clearly men are not immune. In its 2007 publication on eating disorders, the National Institute of Mental Health (NIMH) estimated that 5 to 15 percent of people with anorexia or bulimia and an estimated 35 percent of those with binge-eating disorder are male. Although eating disorders most often appear in the early teen years, they also may occur in young children, the middle-aged, and the elderly.

There are three main types of eating disorders: anorexia, bulimia, and binge-eating disorder. Anorexia is self-imposed starvation and occurs when someone avoids food to the point that he or she is 15 percent or more below a healthy body weight. Bulimia is a disorder in which someone **binges** and then purges. Purging is a way of counteracting overeating through vomiting, excessive exercising, fasting, and/or taking laxatives.

Those who suffer from a binge-eating disorder binge regularly but do not purge. They may or may not be overweight. Many who have the disorder cycle between dieting and bingeing, which keeps them from being **overweight** but does not mean they are healthy. All of these eating disorders are serious mental health problems that should not be ignored. They can and sometimes do cause death.

Now that health experts have learned about eating disorders, some are focusing on prevention, and education is critical. Increasing awareness of eating disorders can help reduce the stigma that may be associated with having one and may increase the number of people who get help early, when treatment has the best chance for success. Efforts to help young people build **self-esteem** by focusing on more than just body image can also go a long way in helping to prevent eating disorders.

TEENAGERS AND THEIR EATING HABITS

This book includes statistics collected as part of the national Youth Risk Behavior Survey published by the Centers for Disease Control and Prevention (CDC) in 2007. The data reveals that many high school students are not as healthy as they could be. Only 21 percent of the students surveyed ate the recommended five or more servings of fruits and vegetables a day. Nearly 41 percent of students said they had eaten less food, fewer calories, or low-fat foods to lose or maintain weight during the month before being surveyed. During the same time period, nearly 12 percent did not eat for a day or more in order to lose or maintain weight.

More than 6 percent of female and nearly 3 percent of male high school students admitted to vomiting or taking laxatives to lose weight or avoid gaining weight. Also, 28.5 percent claimed to have felt "sad or hopeless almost everyday for $\geq$ 2 weeks," which suggests depression, a critical **risk factor** for developing an eating disorder.

EATING DISORDERS IN MEN AND BOYS

While most research has focused on girls and women with eating disorders, eating disorders also affect boys and men. Male interest in athletics may be a cause of some eating disorders, but it is not the only cause. Males, like females, may be prone to eating disorders because of low self-esteem, depression, stress, **anxiety**, or family influence.

Boys and men find more of a stigma attached to eating disorders than girls and women do and therefore may be less likely to seek treatment for the problem. Physicians, friends, and family may also be less inclined to notice the symptoms of eating disorders in boys and men because those illnesses are still more commonly associated with girls and women.

THE SYMPTOMS AND EFFECTS OF EATING DISORDERS

Eating disorders are considered diseases because they have predictable symptoms and outcomes. In fact, there is a long list of symptoms associated with eating disorders. Some of these symptoms are physical and some emotional, while others are related to certain behaviors.

It's not unusual to have a close friend or family member with an eating disorder and not even know it. Even if you spend a lot of time with someone, the signs of an eating disorder can be hard to notice. Not only that, if you do see signs of unusual eating habits or an obvious change in weight in a close friend or family member, you still might have a hard time believing someone close to you has a real problem.

People with eating disorders often go to great lengths to hide their behavior and its effects. Those who have anorexia often wear baggy clothes to camouflage their weight loss. People with bulimia are usually careful to cover the sound of their vomiting with running water and clean up after themselves at home. Binge eaters usually plan their binges at times and in places where they are unlikely to be seen. People with eating disorders may also hide some of the physical symptoms associated with eating disorders, such as fatigue. It is no wonder that detecting an eating disorder in a friend or family member can be so difficult. Still, the more you know about the signs and symptoms of eating disorders, the better prepared you will be to recognize a potential problem either in yourself or someone you care about.

Signs of eating disorders
The Nemours Foundation, ANAD, and other eating-disorders experts list a number of common signs associated with each type of eating disorder. One of the most recognizable and common symptoms of anorexia is a significant amount of weight loss. When anorexia occurs at a young age, when someone is still growing, he or she may not lose any weight at all. For that person, the fact that he or she hasn't gained weight is a symptom of anorexia. Doctors suspecting anorexia look for a patient's weight to be at least 15 percent below his or her healthy body weight.

People with anorexia are often unable to eat very much in a sitting, and they may have stomach pain, heartburn, constipation, and, if they vomit often, tooth decay. They usually feel cold all the time, and may also experience fatigue, dizziness, fainting spells, and **low blood pressure**. (Blood pressure refers to the pressure of the blood on the blood vessels, and when it is lower than normal, it can cause feelings of lightheadedness.) The hair on their head may get thinner and baby fine hair may appear on their face and arms. Female anorexics commonly lose their menstrual periods. Difficulty concentrating and depression are symptoms that also go along with anorexia.

People with bulimia have some of the same symptoms as anorexics, including fatigue, depression, digestive problems that cause stomach pain, heartburn and constipation, and the loss of menstrual periods.

Tooth decay and swollen salivary glands are common symptoms for bulimics because they vomit so often. Anxiety and difficulty sleeping are more symptoms associated with bulimia.

One of the most common symptoms of binge-eating disorder is weight gain. However, sometimes binge-eaters have periods in which they don't overeat and therefore don't have obvious weight gain. Other symptoms associated with binge-eating disorder are stomach pain, internal bleeding, and **high blood pressure**.

Certain behavioral changes may be a sign of an eating disorder. If someone suddenly acquires unusual eating habits, refuses certain foods or types of foods, or eats fewer meals with family and friends, an eating disorder may be the reason. The **compulsive** need to weigh food and measure out portions, the tendency to check weight several times a day, and excessive exercising are other signs of a problem.

Secretive behavior is also a sign of an eating disorder. Often people with eating disorders become alienated from friends and family and ignore everyday activities as they retreat further into their eating, dieting, and exercising rituals.

Body image

Do you care about the way you look? Does it make you feel good about yourself to wear stylish clothes or get a new haircut? Maybe you spend even more time thinking about your clothes, your hair, and your body when you have a romantic interest on the horizon. All of these are perfectly normal behaviors.

It is also normal to sometimes wish you looked or acted a different way. Being a little hard on yourself and thinking you aren't as good as you could be is normal sometimes, too. All of this has to do with your self-image (how you see yourself) and your self-esteem (how you feel about yourself).

Self-image and self-esteem play a large role in eating disorders. One of the main things that people with eating disorders often have in common is a lack of self-esteem. They lack confidence in their value as a person. Body image is central to the way they see themselves and others. They tend to place an abnormally high level of importance on physical appearance and body shape.

An obsession with body image is extremely common in American society and is fueled by the way Americans define beauty and the importance they place on physical beauty. Many studies, including those by Professor Anne Becker of Harvard Medical School, also reveal the influence the media has on self-esteem. These studies suggest that people have more negative feelings about themselves after being bombarded by images of thin celebrities and models—all of whom exhibit an ideal that the average person can't live up to.

A healthy body image requires an understanding that there is no such thing as a "perfect" body, no matter how the term is defined. No one ever achieves perfection. Instead, you can work at feeling good about your body and confident in your movements—strong and graceful rather than clumsy or self-conscious. Such confidence is often the result of healthy eating habits, exercise, and a strong sense of self-esteem that takes into account much more than just body image.

Exercise

Normal exercise habits vary greatly among children and adolescents. Some are actively involved in sports teams. Their participation in regular practices and games gives them a lot of exercise. Some jog, go to the gym, or make some kind of effort to exercise regularly because they want to be fit and healthy. Many teenagers don't make a point to exercise, although they may still get exercise just from being naturally active. Others are either overwhelmed with busy schedules or spend a lot of time doing inactive things, such as watching television or playing video games, and get very little regular exercise.

Is it possible to get too much exercise? The answer is yes. Just as some people exhibit extreme, unhealthy eating habits, people can also have extreme, unhealthy attitudes toward exercise. With all of the emphasis on the importance of exercise, it may be hard to believe that anyone can work out too much. Over-exercising is common among people with anorexia and bulimia. In fact, many **nutritionists** and physicians consider excessive or compulsive exercising a form of purging.

How much exercise is too much? The answer is based more on feelings and actions than on how much time is spent exercising. Exercising is excessive when it dominates your life. For example, if the importance you place on exercise causes you to skip appointments, ignore responsibilities, and/or have little or no time for friends, you may have a problem. If the thought of not exercising for a day makes you feel guilty and anxious, you may be a **compulsive exerciser.**

There is also an eating disorder called bigorexia, or muscle dysmorphia, that is like the opposite of anorexia. Bigorexics exercise excessively in an effort to increase the size of their muscles. However, they never think they look big enough.

If you are a competitive athlete, it may be especially difficult to know at what point your exercise regimen becomes unhealthy. Many athletic pursuits, such as dancing, wrestling, skating, gymnastics, swimming, and cross-country running do put participants at greater risk of having an eating disorder, so it is a good idea to be aware of the possibility and guard against it.

Many compulsive exercisers know they are overdoing their work-out. They often lie about time spent exercising or exercise behind closed doors, using pillows or padding so that no one will hear what they are doing. If any of these actions describe someone you know, he or she has a problem and should get some help.

DIAGNOSING EATING DISORDERS

As hard as it may be to believe that someone close to you might have an eating problem, confronting that person or telling someone else about your suspicions may be even harder. Many people worry that their friend or family member will be angry with them for suggesting they have a problem and need help, and often that is exactly what happens. Someone struggling with an eating disorder may not be open to help from others, but eating disorders are serious problems that need to be dealt with as soon as possible.

Observing symptoms and behaviors is not enough to diagnose an eating disorder. It takes an expert. Those who are suspected of having an eating disorder are generally tested to rule out other reasons for their physical symptoms. They may be given both a physical examination and a psychological test. The standard psychological test used to assess the possibility and the severity of an eating disorder covers these specific areas:

- drive for thinness;
- ineffectiveness (an inability to accomplish things);
- body dissatisfaction;
- interpersonal distrust;
- bulimia;
- perfectionism (the setting of unrealistically high expectations for oneself);
- maturity fear (fear associated with becoming older and more independent, including anxiety about sexual development);

- interoceptive awareness (the ability to identify one's emotions and other internal feelings);
- impulse regulation (the degree to which someone can control his or her urges);
- social insecurity (discomfort caused by social interaction); and
- asceticism (practicing self-denial).

People taking the test are asked to respond to questions using a six-point scale ranging from "always" to "never" and identify their symptoms from a four-page checklist.

THE EFFECTS OF EATING DISORDERS

Eating disorders are life-threatening mental illnesses that can affect not only one's own life but also the lives of loved ones. There is no denying that undergoing treatment for an eating disorder is extremely difficult. The first step is admitting to the problem. Only then can treatment begin. The treatment itself may involve physical discomfort, emotional distress, and the tough job of changing habits. But living with an eating disorder is likely to be more painful, both physically and emotionally.

Physical development

Maturity is something that occurs at different times for different people, so while your friends may show signs of puberty before and after you, in most cases that shouldn't be a cause for concern.

But when eating disorders occur before or around the time of puberty, as they often do, they can slow normal physical and sexual development. An eating disorder may affect a young girl's menstrual cycle, causing a delay in the onset of her first period. If she already has begun menstruation, her periods may become irregular or stop altogether.

Instead of developing hips and breasts, girls with anorexia are likely to have an immature, childlike body shape. Many eating-disorders experts suggest that some people who have these illnesses may be afraid to grow up and become independent or be uncomfortable with the idea of sexual development. Their eating disorder may be a way to avoid maturing and transitioning into a new stage in life.

Social problems

Social situations can be difficult for anyone, and they can be especially hard for people who lack self-confidence. People with eating disorders typically have low self-esteem—one reason they find social situations difficult. When the complexity of an eating disorder is added to low self-esteem, social problems become even more pronounced.

Think about how often social activities involve food. If someone who binges loses control when confronted by large amounts of food, Thanksgiving at Grandma's is extremely stressful. So is a party with lots of junk food at a friend's house. Those who have anorexia often don't want people to know how little they eat, so they may avoid eating in public. For those with bulimia, a weekend trip may be out of the question simply because the opportunities to purge may be limited.

Even if food was not central to many social situations, an eating disorder would still hamper healthy relationships with friends and family. As the disorder progresses, it is likely to take up more and more space in one's life, crowding out other things—including friendships. Instead of planning something special for a friend's birthday, those with an eating disorder may calculate how many **calories** they've exercised off today and how to get some more exercise in. Also, it is hard to be a good friend when you're tired, depressed, moody, and anxious.

Health problems

If you have ever seen a picture of someone with anorexia, it's not hard to believe that he or she is malnourished. Those who have bulimia or binge can also be malnourished. They may consume a lot of food, but those foods rarely have the vitamins and minerals they need to keep their bodies healthy.

Other problems caused by eating disorders include **dehydration**, kidney problems, stomach damage, low blood pressure, and heart problems. Those who binge and become obese are at risk of **diabetes**, heart attack, **stroke**, and even a fatal stomach rupture. Compulsive exercising adds more health problems. Instead of building muscles, too much exercise can destroy them. Overexercising can cause physical problems, such as dehydration, broken bones, joint problems, osteoporosis, and **organ failure**.

Every type of eating disorder is potentially deadly. Many people with eating disorders die of organ failure. Others commit **suicide**. Severe depression sometimes leads to suicide, and many people who have eating disorders also suffer from depression. According to the National Institute of Mental Health (NIMH), between 6 and 8.3 percent of all adolescents have suicidal thoughts, which often go unrecognized and untreated.

Long-term effects

When eating disorders go untreated, health problems become more and more severe and life threatening. Those who do not get treatment for their eating disorder are 10 times more likely to die from that disorder than if they received treatment.

Treatment doesn't guarantee recovery. Anorexia Nervosa and Related Eating Disorders, Incorporated (ANRED) reports that about 20 percent of those who get treatment fail to make a full recovery and continue to wrestle with food issues or relapse. Another 20 percent are unable to overcome their eating disorders. The earlier a disorder is treated, the better one's chances of recovery.

WHAT ARE THE NUMBERS?

Although evidence shows that eating disorders have existed for hundreds of years, the study of eating disorders is still a relatively new field. Statistics are constantly changing. Recovery rates are hard to quantify, because the length of the recovery period can vary significantly. It may take five years before someone can be considered well. A 2005 study published in the *European Eating Disorders Review* tracked more than 600 patients and found that after two and a half years, more than 32 percent of the patients with anorexia and more than 37 percent of the patients with bulimia had relapsed. The patients' highest risk of relapse occurred about six months after they had at least partially overcome their eating disorders.

RISKY BUSINESS SELF-TEST

Some people with eating disorders deny that they have a problem. Others are aware that something is wrong but try to hide it. Still other people believe that they are in control of their eating disorder and therefore it isn't a problem. To identify whether you have a problem or are at risk for an eating disorder, record your answers to this short true-or-false test on a sheet of paper.

A. The first set of statements deal with body image:

1. I care a lot about the way my body looks, and I am never satisfied with how it looks.

    2. People tell me I'm thin, but I don't believe them.

    3. I would be happier if I looked like the models on TV and in magazines.

    4. When I see people who are thinner than I am, particularly models and celebrities in the media, I feel bad about the way I look.

B. The second set of statements addresses factors that may increase the risk of an eating disorder:

    1. People who play important roles in my life are verbally abusive—constantly criticizing my appearance.

    2. I have been sexually or physically abused.

    3. Someone in my immediate family has or had an eating disorder.

    4. I often feel depressed, and my depression affects how much I eat.

C. The final set of statements deals with behaviors:

    1. I am constantly trying to diet.

    2. I always keep track of how many calories and how many **fats** I am consuming.

    3. I weigh myself more than once a day.

    4. I am willing to take risks to lose weight.

    5. I am willing to take risks to become stronger.

    6. I sometimes vomit because I eat too much.

    7. I have to lose weight to participate in sports or dance.

    8. I have experimented with weight-loss drugs, laxatives, and/or **diuretics.**

    9. I am secretive about the amount of food I eat and/or the amount of time I spend exercising.

    10. It makes me feel strong when I can resist the urge to eat for long periods of time.

    11. I eat large quantities of food and then feel bad about myself.

12. My eating and/or exercise habits often keep me from participating in social activities or fulfilling my responsibilities.

Scoring

Part A: Answering true to any one of the four statements means that you are not comfortable with the way your body looks, and you are at some risk of developing an eating disorder.

Part B: If you answer true to any of these statements, there are factors in your life that increase your likelihood of getting an eating disorder.

Part C: Answering true to any of these statements means you are exhibiting unhealthy behaviors that are often seen among people who have eating disorders. You should seek help in order to stop these behaviors.

If you think you may have an eating disorder, you should never be ashamed to talk about it with someone you trust, or at the very least, read up on the subject. There is a wealth of information on eating disorders and healthy eating in this book, in the library, and on the Web. Gathering information is a great first step. After that, it is easier to be open with others and get the help you or someone you know may need.

A TO Z ENTRIES

■ ANOREXIA

Self-imposed starvation. Like all eating disorders, it is considered a mental illness that can cause severe physical problems. The most worrisome thing about anorexia is that it's a killer. In fact, it has one of the highest mortality (death) rates of any mental illness.

You might not have realized that anorexia is a form of mental illness, but it is. Emotional issues are typically at the root of the disorder.

Most of the statistics on anorexia focus on young women, since they are the group most likely to develop the eating disorder. The National Institute of Mental Health (NIMH) reports that young women between the ages of 15 and 24 who have anorexia have a 12 times greater chance of dying at their young age than friends of the same age—higher than any other cause of death among females of that age group. Many of the deaths attributed to anorexia are **suicides**, but the physical problems caused by the disorder—esophageal rupture, heart failure, and **stroke**—can also be deadly.

WHO GETS ANOREXIA?

Although anorexia affects people of all ages, genders, and ethnic backgrounds, the people most likely to develop the eating disorder are young Caucasian women who are high academic achievers and have a goal-oriented family or personality. A survey published in 2007 in *Biological Psychiatry* found that 0.9 percent of women and 0.3 percent of men had had anorexia some time during their lives.

Q & A

Question: My boyfriend lost a lot of weight while training for a gymnastics competition. The competition is over and he's still exercising constantly and eating very few calories. My mom says I'm worrying over nothing because she's never heard of a guy having anorexia. Is she right?

Answer: Even though males are less likely than females to get anorexia, it does happen. In fact, the National Institute of Mental Health reported in 2007 that one in four preadolescent cases of anorexia occurs in boys. So if you suspect your boyfriend has a problem, don't ignore it.

By middle school, young people are at that odd stage in life where they feel that they are neither children nor adults. By high school that feeling has intensified. They have become more independent but are still expected to live by their parents' rules.

Some teens resent their parents for placing too many restrictions on them. Others have families with serious emotional problems, such as abuse or **addiction**. Both groups recognize that one thing parents can't do is force their children to eat. Therefore, a number of teens may decide not to eat as a way of gaining a sense of control over their life.

Still other teenagers believe that they will never live up to their own or their parents' expectations about their appearance, popularity, or ability to succeed in sports, academics, or the arts. So they deny themselves the pleasure of eating as a means of punishment.

Some teens are afraid of growing up and taking complete responsibility for their lives. The prospect of increasing independence makes them feel out of control. Not eating helps them gain a sense of control, even though just the opposite is true. As anorexia progresses, it takes total control.

Fact Or Fiction?

Mothers are too old to have anorexia.

The Facts: Although anorexia usually starts at a young age, it can appear at any age. Some people suffer with anorexia for decades. The NIH reports that women who develop and deal with anorexia at an early age have a better chance of complete recovery. According to the National Association of Anorexia Nervosa and Associated Disorders (ANAD), the longer someone lives with anorexia, the greater the chance he or she may die from it.

WARNING SIGNS AND HEALTH PROBLEMS ASSOCIATED WITH ANOREXIA

Those who suffer from anorexia have a distorted body image and an overwhelming fear of gaining weight. These are some of the warning signs of the eating disorder:

- weight loss of 15 percent or more below the ideal body weight;
- dieting, when not **overweight**;

- perceiving oneself as fat;

- exercising excessively;

- being preoccupied with food, dieting, and nutrition;

- feeling nauseous or bloated after eating small amounts of food;

- loss of hair; and

- in the case of women, not menstruating.

Very often, those who experience the extreme weight loss that characterizes anorexia may be hospitalized. By that time, they also may be experiencing a wide range of related health problems. Anorexia taxes the central nervous system, making it difficult to think and concentrate. People with anorexia are apt to be tired, listless, and depressed. Their hair thins. They may start to see fine hair on their face and arms, like babies have.

You may have heard parents tell children that they need to eat healthy foods to grow big and strong. It's true. Anorexia can stunt growth and cause osteoporosis, a progressive loss of bone density. Sexual development also may be stunted and girls may stop having their period.

Anorexia places severe strain on the organs. Kidney problems are common, as are heart problems. The pulse may be slow and become irregular. Blood pressure may drop, which can make a person feel dizzy or faint easily. People with anorexia get cold easily, and their lips and fingers may turn blue. They may experience chest pain, and in the worst cases, die from cardiac arrest. The list of health problems goes on to include stomach pains, heartburn, constipation, and dental problems—especially for those who vomit often.

Fact Or Fiction?

You can never lose enough weight.

The Facts: People suffering from anorexia look in the mirror and what they see is never good enough. Their friends and family may say they look too thin, but they don't think that's possible. They may look in the mirror and "see" fat where there is none. They typically like to see their bones sticking out.

The idea that it is impossible to be "too thin" is not just wrong, it is deadly. When people fall too far below their ideal body weight, they lose their ability to concentrate and remember things, lack energy, and eventually encounter severe health problems due to organ failure.

Q & A

Question: Is it possible to have anorexia without losing a lot of weight?

Answer: It sounds odd, but someone can have anorexia without any loss of weight. Children who are still growing are expected to increase their body weight. If they diet during those years and grow taller without gaining weight, they may drop below 85 percent of the healthy body weight for the new height and, in that case, be diagnosed with anorexia.

TREATING ANOREXIA

One of the biggest challenges in treating anorexia is the fact that most people who suffer from it are in denial. They don't believe they are underweight or engaged in dangerous eating habits. For that reason, diagnosing the eating disorder in its early stages can be difficult.

To figure out if someone is suffering from the eating disorder, doctors run tests to determine whether physical problems may be causing **unintentional weight loss**. Once anorexia is diagnosed, both the physical and emotional issues must be treated. The first objective is to increase the patient's body weight to a healthier range, improve eating habits, and address related physical problems. If the patient's body weight is 30 percent below normal, he or she is likely to be hospitalized and may even need intravenous feeding.

Emotional issues may be treated with **psychotherapy, behavioral therapy, support groups,** and **antidepressant** drug therapy. Psychotherapy involves talking with a therapist to figure out the causes and extent of one's emotional problems. Behavioral therapy is a way of trying to modify behavior through reward or punishment. In support groups, people dealing with similar problems help each other get better. With antidepressant drug therapy, a physician prescribes medication that can help a patient with the physical and emotional symptoms of depression, such as poor sleep, low energy, difficulty concentrating, low self-esteem, and inability to feel pleasure.

Unfortunately, anorexia is not easily cured. A 15-year survival study published in 1997 by the *International Journal of Eating Disorders* and a 10-year survival study published in 1995 by *Psychological Medicine* showed that 30 to 50 percent of patients treated successfully in the hospital become ill again within one year of leaving the hospital. A number of researchers are experimenting with treatment programs that may prevent **relapses**. A 1998 study published by *Clinical Psychology Review* found that a kind of psychotherapy known as **cognitive-behavioral therapy**, which tries to change a person's attitudes in order to change their behaviors, can lower relapse rates. In 2004, a study at Toronto General Hospital had a similar result, with a 35 percent relapse rate, with the highest risk occurring six to 17 months after discharge.

Q & A

Question: My friend has many of the warning signs of anorexia. When I try to talk to her about it, she just won't listen. How can I help her?

Answer: Drop the subject for a while because she needs your friendship. In the meantime, mention your concerns to her parents, teachers, and anyone else you think she respects. You never know who might get through to her. You can also discuss your concerns with an expert in eating disorders. Try ANAD's toll-free hotline Monday through Friday from 10 a.m. to 6 p.m. Eastern Time at 847–831–3438 or find them on the Web at www.anad.org.

TEENS SPEAK

I Hated Myself Because I Thought I Was Fat

My senior year in high school, I was in the honor society, played field hockey, and had lots of friends. You never would have thought anything was wrong, but I hated myself because I thought I was fat. I thought I'd never have a boyfriend or be truly happy unless I was thin.

It wasn't long before I became compulsive about counting calories. I carefully planned what I would eat for the week, skipping meals and exercising excessively whenever I thought I'd consumed too many calories. I took up to six laxatives a day. Even though I really missed eating the foods I used to love, it was all worth it when I'd get on the scale and see I had lost more weight.

Friends would say how lucky I was to be thin, even though my period stopped, my hair fell out, and my face became wan and swollen. I used to count my ribs lying in bed at night.

Ironically, even though my anorexia started with a desire to attract boys, it soon made me lose interest in them. I couldn't stand the thought of someone getting close enough to me to look at or touch my body. I had one girlfriend who was really worried about me, but I refused to believe I had a problem. When my field hockey coach said that she thought I had a problem, I took it to heart but felt paralyzed and couldn't help myself.

One day I blacked out and ended up in the hospital. There was no avoiding that I was an anorexic. In the hospital, my mother was actually shocked to see how underweight I was. She used to be jealous of the "cute, skinny jeans" I could wear.

The most important part of my recovery was emotional. My whole family went into therapy. My mother and I, in particular, worked hard to understand why my self-esteem was so low and how to improve it. Unfortunately, I can't say the story ends there. My junior year in college I had a relapse. But that time, the signs were easier to recognize and I got help. It was like reliving an awful nightmare. But I got better.

I look back and realize how much I used to lie to hide my anorexia. I don't know that I can say I'm perfectly well now, but I have stopped lying. Being open about what I've been through helps me stay true to myself and feel more confident about who I am, inside and out.

IS IT REALLY ANOREXIA?

Skipping a meal here and there is not healthy, but it is not anorexia. Anorexia fills up a person's life and takes control of it. Food and dieting become an obsession that can last a lifetime if not treated. Even after people with anorexia have recovered, they are likely to struggle with negative feelings about food and body fat. The warning signs of anorexia may not always be obvious, but if you detect them, they should never be ignored.

See also: Depression and Weight; Eating Disorders, Causes of; Eating Disorders, Symptoms and Diagnosis of; Media and Eating Disorders; Morbidity and Mortality; Nutrition and Nutritional Deficiencies; Treatment; Women and Eating Disorders

FURTHER READING

Levenkron, Steven. *Anatomy of Anorexia*. New York: W. W. Norton & Company, 2001.
National Institute of Mental Health. "Study Tracks Prevalence of Eating Disorders." National Institute of Mental Health: Science News. URL: http://www.nimh.nih.gov/science-news/2007/study-tracks-prevalence-of-eating-disorders.shtml. Posted February 9, 2007.
Sullivan, P. F. "Mortality in Anorexia Nervosa." *American Journal of Psychiatry* 152, no. 7 (1995): 1,073–1,074.

■ BIGOREXIA/MUSCLE DYSMORPHIA

A preoccupation or obsession with being muscular. Most people look at themselves sometimes and think they could look better. Guys, in particular, often think they should have bigger muscles.

There is no great secret to becoming more muscular. It takes exercise. Many people begin an exercise regimen as teenagers. They go to the gym regularly and lift weights and feel good about their bodies. Exercise makes you feel strong and relatively attractive. That's perfectly healthy.

Bigorexia, however, is a much different condition. It has to do with what your body actually looks like and the way you perceive your body. Think of bigorexia as the opposite of anorexia. While anorexics look in a mirror and despair that they are not thinner and smaller, bigorexics see someone scrawny and weak and wish they looked stronger and more muscular.

Just as is the case with anorexia, the way bigorexics see themselves is usually not what is actually reflected in the mirror. Even as they work out and build up their muscles, those with bigorexia see their bodies as the enemy—finding flaws where there are none and feeling this drive to create bigger and more impressive muscles.

IDENTIFYING MUSCLE DYSMORPHIA

A more scientific term for bigorexia is **muscle dysmorphia**. The study of muscle dysmorphia is relatively new. In 1993, Harrison Pope, Jr., a leading psychiatric researcher at Harvard, and his colleagues were studying anabolic steroid use among weightlifters and in the course of that research identified something they called reverse anorexia nervosa. They found striking similarities between anorexia and reverse anorexia, including compulsive and ritualistic behavior, excessive exercise, and dissatisfaction with one's body to the point of wanting to hide in baggy clothes.

Later, Pope and his colleagues suggested that reverse anorexia nervosa be referred to, instead, as muscle dysmorphia and be considered a form of **body dysmorphic disorder**.

People with body dysmorphic disorder are so preoccupied with an imagined problem in their physical appearance that their everyday lives are impacted. The term *muscle dysmorphia* has stuck, but where it should be classified among psychiatric disorders is still being debated. Some researchers believe that both body dysmorphic disorder and muscle dysmorphia should be classified as **obsessive-compulsive disorders**.

However it is classified, muscle dysmorphia is clearly centered around body image. In 2000, Pope coauthored a book called *The Adonis Complex: The Secret Crisis of Male Body Obsession* and brought more attention to the issue.

Pope and his coauthors write about how the media and other cultural influences present an ideal body image for men that is unrealistic and largely impossible to achieve in a healthy way. Muscle dysmorphia is just one of the unhealthy behaviors that boys and men may develop as they strive to improve their physical appearance.

WHO GETS BIGOREXIA?

Muscle dysmorphia, or bigorexia, is not strictly a male disorder, but it is believed to affect more men than women. Low self-esteem, media and cultural influences, and peer pressure all contribute to bigorexia.

In 2005, a writer for the *International Journal of Men's Health* reviewed studies from 1997, 2000, and 2001 and determined that the mean age of onset for muscle dysmorphia is just over 19 years old. In November 2007, a CBS-TV news station reported that bigorexia is a growing problem that affects hundreds of thousands of men and women.

Why is the trend growing?

A 2006 survey published in the *Canadian Journal of Psychiatry* found that men's dissatisfaction with their bodies has increased dramatically in the last 30 years. American culture seems to glorify the muscular male body just as it does the thin female figure. Just as unrealistically skinny Barbie dolls marketed to little girls are associated with anorexia, bulked-up GI Joe action figures marketed to boys are associated with bigorexia. At http://www.brainphysics.com/muscle-dysmorphia.php, you can look at pictures of GI Joe from the 1960s and GI Joe today. The muscles on today's GI Joe are not only bigger but much more defined.

On store shelves, you can also find more fitness magazines than ever before. While many promote healthy lifestyles, the proliferation of these magazines means men and women are bombarded with more images of buff bodies to aspire to.

Q & A

Question: I have been telling my parents not to worry about the amount of time I spend exercising, but they aren't convinced. How can we be sure that my regimen is safe?

Answer: ANRED recommends that you start by getting evaluated by a general physician. You should always consult a doctor before beginning an exercise routine. If you are at a healthy weight, an appropriate routine should make you feel good. However, if the doctor feels you have a problem, you also should be evaluated by a mental health counselor who has experience with muscle dysmorphia. If you are diagnosed with muscle dysmorphia, **cognitive behavioral therapy** and medication are likely to be recommended to help you.

DANGERS OF BIGOREXIA

Lifting weights and exercising is healthy; however, taking it to extremes and obsessing over the size of your muscles can be extremely unhealthy.

According to Anorexia Nervosa and Related Eating Disorders, Inc. (ANRED), people with muscle dysmorphia tend to also suffer from depression, and their self-consciousness about their appearance takes a toll on school, work, and personal relationships. The more time you spend in the gym or lifting weights at home, the less time you will have for normal activities, such as studying or socializing.

It is typical for bigorexics to continue lifting weights even when they are injured, an obviously dangerous habit. Of most concern, though, is the potential for drug addiction. What bigorexics see as the ideal image is often unattainable without the "help" of drugs that can seriously endanger their health, or even kill them.

Bigorexia and drug use

Anabolic steroids include natural substances that your body makes, as well as medications that doctors prescribe for specific medical conditions. It is illegal to take these drugs to improve athletic performance or increase muscle size, but that has not stopped many bodybuilders and other athletes from trying them and becoming addicted.

The National Institute on Drug Abuse (NIDA), a branch of the National Institutes of Health (NIH), cites these "major side effects" caused by anabolic steroids: liver tumors, cancer, jaundice, fluid retention, high blood pressure, increases in LDL (the "bad" cholesterol), and decreases in HDL (the "good" cholesterol). They also list kidney tumors, severe acne, and trembling as possible side effects, which may not technically qualify as "major" but are serious enough for most people, especially teens.

Because steroids are related to male sex hormones, they also have side effects that are gender-specific. Men who take steroids can end up with fertility problems, lose their hair, and grow breasts. Women's voices can get deeper, and they can grow facial hair and experience male-pattern baldness when taking steroids.

Fact Or Fiction

Taking steroids can stunt your growth.

The Facts: Using steroids when you are not under a doctor's supervision is especially dangerous to teenagers. During adolescence, steroids can stop your bones from growing and accelerate the onset of puberty. That means that if you take anabolic steroids before your growth spurt, you may never grow as tall as you were meant to be.

DID YOU KNOW?

Students Who Have Used Anabolic Steroids at Least Once in Their Lifetime

8th Grade	10th Grade	12th Grade
1.6%	1.8%	2.7%

Source: National Institute on Drug Abuse, 2006 Monitoring the Future Survey.

Perhaps as a result of increased awareness of these side effects, steroid use among teenagers is down. NIDA conducts regular surveys on drug use among eighth, 10th, and 12th grade students. Their news is good. In 2006 less than 2 percent of eighth and 10th graders and less than 3 percent of 12th graders had used steroids at least once during their lifetime.

DISTORTED IMAGES

Do you have a friend who is constantly asking you if he is bigger than other guys you see at the gym? ANRED says that when bigorexics ask people how their body looks, it's because their mind finds it difficult to understand what their body really looks like. In other words, they aren't just fishing for compliments—they really don't see what you see.

See also: Eating Disorders in Men and Boys; Exercise

FURTHER READING

Luciano, Lynne. *Looking Good: Male Body Image in Modern America.* New York: Hill and Wang, 2002.

Pope, Harrison G., Jr., Katharine A. Phillips, and Roberto Olivardia. *The Adonis Complex: The Secret Crisis of Male Body Obsession.* New York: Free Press, 2002.

■ BINGE-EATING DISORDER

A mental condition in which a person periodically consumes huge amounts of food in a short period of time. Binge-eating disorder is very similar to bulimia, except that bulimics purge after they overeat and binge-eaters do not.

Binge eating is not the same as overeating. Almost everyone over-eats on occasion. Overeating is when you indulge in that second or even third helping of your favorite dessert once in a while. Or when you split a pizza with some friends after studying, even though you really aren't hungry.

Binge eating is very different. If you were having an actual binge-eating episode, you would feel completely unable to control your eating, to the extent that you might not even notice what you are eating or how it tastes. You would feel full and keep eating. Your stomach would hurt, but that would not stop you either. Afterward, you would feel terrible about what you had done, but it would happen again another day, and another day after that. Each time you had the urge to **binge**, you would feel totally unable to stop yourself.

Just as overeating is different from bingeing, bingeing one time does not mean you have an eating disorder. Diagnostic criteria established by the American Psychiatric Association (APA) says that those with the disorder binge, on average, twice a week for at least six months.

Eating so much food so quickly is painful, both physically and emotionally. Sometimes, binge-eaters are referred to as compulsive eaters or food addicts.

You might expect that someone who binges regularly would be extremely overweight and easy to spot, but that is not necessarily the case. Some binge-eaters keep their weight under control by diet-ing between binges. Even though they may fall into a healthy weight range on a chart, those binge-eaters are not healthy.

Other binge-eaters, though, do gain weight from their excessive overeating. They are likely to be **obese**, with an unhealthy amount of body fat, which puts them at risk for many serious health problems.

TEENS SPEAK

Cookies Under My Bed

When I was little, my mom was always onto me about mak-ing my bed and cleaning my room. Now that I'm older, she thinks her lectures have sunk in. She never has to remind me to make my bed or clean my room. She doesn't know that I keep it so clean to keep her from poking around.

Now instead of worrying about my room, she worries about my wallet. "What do you do with all your money?" she keeps asking me. I can't tell my mom the real answer, so I mumble something about expensive coffee and music downloads.

The truth is that I spend my money at the grocery store. Cookies, chips, and candy—it's amazing how they can add up. I stay away from name brands, choosing whatever's least expensive or on sale, or both. I want my money to equal as much junk food as possible.

I sneak the food in when my parents are at work and hide it under my bed. Now you see why I've become such a neat freak. If my mother, who is always talking about nutrition and healthy habits, found my stash, she would go crazy. She already worries that I don't eat breakfast before school. But mornings are a mad rush and I never have time.

School is a nightmare. Every day. I've been the new kid for three years now. Moving to a town where everyone has been friends since kindergarten is just as bad as every chapter book you ever read in elementary school portrays it to be. The books always have happy endings though. I'm still waiting for that part. Until then, at least I have the food under my bed.

It's sort of funny that knowing there's food under my bed makes me feel better, since eating it makes me feel terrible. Last night I finished everything that was under there. I had waited until my parents were asleep. My music was on, as always, so they couldn't hear the packages crinkling. I finished a bag of chips and a box of cookies in about 15 minutes and I can't even remember what kind they were. All I know is that they were both family-sized packages.

My stomach hurt afterward. And I felt horribly guilty. Yesterday was supposed to be the day I stopped all this crazy eating. After every binge, I lie in bed, feeling guilty, and make that same promise to myself. That I'll stop. I know it's bad for me. But it's such an overwhelming feeling, when I pull the food out from under my bed. I just can't stop myself from ripping into the packages, and eating until there's nothing left but crumbs.

WHO GETS BINGE-EATING DISORDER?

A study published in *Biological Psychiatry* in February 2007 found that of the three major eating disorders, binge eating was the most common. The researchers, led by James I. Hudson of McLean Hospital and Harvard Medical School, looked at survey data from nearly 3,000 adults collected between February 2001 and December 2003 as part of the National Institute of Mental Health (NIMH)–funded National Comorbidity Survey Replication. They found that 3.5 percent of women and 2 percent of men had suffered from binge-eating disorder at some point in their lives, more than the number of people reporting that they suffered from anorexia (0.9 percent of women and 0.3 percent of men) or bulimia (1.5 percent of women and 0.5 percent of men).

Previous studies found similar results. In its *Numbers Count 2006*, NIMH reports that binge-eating disorder affects between 2 percent and 5 percent of Americans, and that 35 percent of them are male, citing studies done in the early 1990s. Estimates on the total population affected by binge-eating disorder vary, but all estimates show it to be the most prevalent eating disorder in the nation.

Anorexia Nervosa and Related Eating Disorders, Inc. (ANRED) reports that 30 percent of women who seek out professional weight loss treatment binge, and ANRED estimates that 1 to 2 million adult Americans struggle with bingeing. The Weight-control Information Network (WIN), a service of the National Institute of Diabetes and Digestive and Kidney Diseases, reports that as many as 4 million Americans have the disorder. It seems to be especially common among obese people, according to WIN and other research groups.

Unlike other eating disorders, WIN reports that binge-eating disorder is most common among adults between the ages of 46 and 55 years. WIN also also reports a similar incidence of binge-eating disorder among blacks and whites; studies have not been done on the prevalence of the disorder among other ethnic groups.

WARNING SIGNS AND HEALTH PROBLEMS ASSOCIATED WITH BINGE-EATING DISORDER

The National Eating Disorders Association (NEDA) lists the following as indicators of binge-eating disorder:

- frequent episodes of eating large quantities of food in short periods of time
- feeling out of control over eating behavior

- feeling ashamed or disgusted by the behavior
- eating when not hungry
- eating in secret

As anyone who has ever overeaten can imagine, a binge episode can cause stomach pain. The more often you binge, the more pain you're likely to endure. However, there are also health problems associated with binge eating that are much more serious, with chronic and even life-threatening consequences. According to NEDA, they are:

- high blood pressure
- high cholesterol levels
- heart disease
- diabetes
- gallbladder disease

These symptoms, as you might recognize, are also associated with obesity, which is considered by many experts to be an American health epidemic.

Q & A

Question: If binge-eaters are secretive about their habits, how will I know if a friend is having a problem?

Answer: As binge-eaters learn that they are not alone, they are more likely to seek treatment. If your friend won't talk about his or her eating habits, has gained otherwise unexplained weight, and appears depressed, he or she may have binge-eating disorder.

TREATING BINGE-EATING DISORDER

The fact that most binge-eaters have their bingeing episodes in secret compounds their problem. They hide what they're doing out of shame and guilt, and that means you might not be able to recognize that someone is suffering from the disorder. This can make it take longer for them to get help.

Binge-eaters typically punish their bodies for a long time. In James Hudson's study, he found that people who were binge-eaters generally had the condition for about eight years. NEDA and others make it clear that binge eating is an emotional disorder, often accompanied by depression, distress, shame, and guilt. For that reason, the American Psychiatric Association says that treatment must go beyond an effort to stop the compulsion to binge and focus on the underlying feelings and thoughts that trigger the binge-eating behavior. The association recommends a combination of medical care, nutritional counseling, psychotherapy, and in some cases medication.

Binge-eaters often suffer alone and in silence. But WIN stresses the importance of spreading the word that binge eating is not uncommon and that most people who struggle with it aren't successful in controlling it on their own. Most people require treatment, but if they get it, they are likely to get better.

WHY DO PEOPLE BINGE?

Most researchers believe that bingeing is a response to stress, anxiety, anger, and other emotions that the binge-eater is having trouble handling. People who binge tend to have certain behaviors and feelings in common. They may abuse alcohol, act impulsively, feel out of control in their lives, feel disconnected from their communities, and keep their emotions to themselves, according to WIN.

Binge eating has also been reported to occur among several people in the same family. Researchers are just starting to look at whether genetics play a factor in binge eating.

Biological factors can cause overeating, too, according to The Nemours Foundation's Center for Children's Health Media. (Nemours has an informative Web site called TeensHealth: http://www.kidshealth.org/teen.) Overeating can result when your **hypothalamus** (the part of your brain that controls hunger) does not send a signal through your brain that you are full or when you do not have the right amount of **serotonin**, a chemical in your brain that affects your mood.

Q & A

Question: Are the cravings women have during pregnancy related to binge-eating disorder?

Answer: Cravings during pregnancy are normal and aren't the same as binge eating, which is characterized by eating very large quantities of food very quickly and often in secret. But there could be a link between pregnancy and binge-eating disorder.

In August 2007, researchers at the University of North Carolina at Chapel Hill studying 100,000 pregnant Norwegian women announced that they were surprised to find an increase in the onset of binge-eating disorder during pregnancy, and that bingeing was more likely to continue than not among the women who were already binge-eaters when they got pregnant. Cynthia M. Bulik is leading the research and now hopes to study how the binge eating during pregnancy has affected the women's offspring.

BINGE EATING AND DEPRESSION

Binge-eating disorder has not been studied as long or as extensively as other eating disorders, so researchers are still looking for answers. Most of the literature on binge eating mentions depression. WIN reports that half of the people suffering from binge-eating disorder are or have been depressed. The mystery is whether the depression or the eating disorder comes first, and no one has the definitive answer yet.

See also: Bulimia; Eating Disorders, Symptoms and Diagnosis of; Obesity

FURTHER READING

Danowski, Debbie, Ph.D. *Locked Up for Eating Too Much: The Diary of a Food Addict in Rehab.* Center City, Minn.: Hazelden, 2002.
Weight-control Information Network. *Binge Eating Disorder.* NIH Publication No. 04-3589. Bethesda, Md.: September 2004.
Nemours Foundation. "Binge Eating Disorder," TeensHealth. URL: http://www.kidshealth.org/teen/food_fitness/problems/binge_eating.html. Updated July 2006.

■ BODY IMAGE

See: Anorexia; Media and Eating Disorders; Peer Pressure; Self-Image

■ BULIMIA

A mental disorder characterized by overeating followed by purging. Those who have bulimia are suffering from what can be a deadly cycle. The American Psychiatric Association classifies people who **binge** (engage in uncontrolled eating) and purge, on average, at least twice a week for three months as having bulimia. Purging is an attempt to erase the consequences of a binge by vomiting, using laxatives or diuretics, or even exercising obsessively.

A famous commercial shows a man who has just eaten a gluttonous meal. He groans, "I can't believe I ate the whole thing!" In the commercial, all it takes are two fizzy antacid tablets to make him feel better. People with bulimia start out much like the man in the commercial. They too are looking for easy relief for their discomfort, but they have more than a bad case of heartburn. Their discomfort comes from a binge—not just a big meal.

A person with bulimia may feel helpless, depressed, or anxious. Binge eating and purging may be an attempt to gain some control in life. In reality, bulimia is a sign that someone has lost control. It's not unusual for someone with bulimia to feel out of control in many other areas of life as well. The person who struggles with bulimia may also be prone to **compulsive** spending, drug or alcohol abuse, or unhealthy relationships.

Q & A

Question: The last time I spent the night at my girlfriend's house, I brought over some sugar wafers. We stayed up late and by the end of the night we had eaten the whole package. I didn't throw up but I did feel kind of sick. Is that what a binge is like?

Answer: No. A binge is much more intense. When someone has a true binge, he or she experiences a total lack of control. Often, that person is preoccupied with thoughts of food before the binge. During the binge itself, the person eats unusually quickly and a lot more than half a package of cookies. She may or may not feel full even after eating a huge quantity of food. After a binge, a bulimic typically feels disgusted by his or her behavior. The reaction to purging is usually different. Instead of disgust, those with bulimia often feel relieved and cleansed.

WHO GETS BULIMIA?

Even though many more women than men suffer from the eating disorder, bulimia is by no means a female disorder. Researchers find one male with bulimia for every 10 to 15 females, according to a study published in the *American Journal of Psychiatry* in April 2001. And results of a large, national survey published in *Biological Psychiatry* in 2007 found that 1.5 percent of women and 0.5 percent of men said they had been bulimic.

People with bulimia are usually very concerned with their weight and may feel dissatisfied with their bodies. Athletes who compete in sports that place a strong emphasis on weight—including wrestling, ballet, ice skating, and gymnastics—sometimes develop bulimia.

The Youth Risk Behavior Survey, conducted in 2007, asked high school students about the different ways in which they had tried to lose weight or keep from gaining weight during the thirty days before the survey. Sixty percent had exercised and more than 40 percent had chosen foods based on low calorie or fat content. A much smaller percentage chose more radical methods, which included fasting, vomiting, or taking diet pills.

WARNING SIGNS AND HEALTH PROBLEMS ASSOCIATED WITH BULIMIA

People with bulimia can sometimes be hard to spot, because their weight is likely to remain unchanged. Even though bulimia is not characterized by a dramatic weight loss, it can be just as damaging

DID YOU KNOW?

How High School Students Tried to Lose or Avoid Gaining Weight

	Exercised	Ate less, fewer calories, or foods low in fat	Fasted for more than 24 hours	Took diet aids	Vomited or took laxatives
Female	67.0%	53.2%	16.3%	7.5%	6.4%
Male	65.0%	28.3%	7.3%	4.2%	2.2%

Source: Youth Risk Behavior Survey, 2007.

to one's health as anorexia. Experts say the most common signs that someone is suffering from bulimia include:

- a preoccupation with food;
- overeating as a reaction to emotional stress;
- the consumption of huge amounts of food without gaining weight;
- frequent use of the bathroom after meals;
- compulsive exercise;
- swollen cheeks; and
- broken blood vessels in the eyes.

Fact Or Fiction?

It's important to keep my weight within the ideal range for my height, no matter what.

The Facts: There is no such thing as an ideal weight. There is, however, a healthy weight range. You can determine a healthy weight range for your height by consulting a Body Mass Index (BMI) chart. Keep in mind that how that weight is maintained is also important. Bingeing and purging to control weight is unhealthy. Your "healthy weight range" is only as healthy as the eating habits used to maintain it.

Other warning signals may be especially hard to detect, because they involve actions that are carried out in private. For example, someone with bulimia is likely to:

- binge secretly, without the ability to stop voluntarily;
- vomit after binge eating; and
- abuse laxatives, diuretics, and diet pills.

Q & A

Question: Is bulimia really bad for you?

Answer: People with anorexia look as if they are starving, so it's easier to tell that they are unhealthy. People with bulimia may be in a healthy weight range for their height, but looks can be deceiving. Bingeing and purging can leave a person's body with so few nutrients that he or she may be starving, even if his or her weight doesn't change. Vomiting, using laxatives, and exercising excessively cause many other health problems. Bulimia also takes a toll on your mental health, making a person more depressed as he or she sinks deeper into his or her own world.

Many of the health problems associated with bulimia come from purging. Vomiting brings up stomach acid, which can cause serious tooth decay, swollen salivary glands (which is why someone's cheeks may look swollen), and the loss of a dangerous amount of potassium. Low levels of potassium levels can result in fatal heart problems.

Like anorexia, bulimia places stress on the body's organs. Bulimia can damage the stomach and kidneys, causing constant stomach pain. Girls may also stop menstruating, due to abnormal **hormone** levels.

Q & A

Question: My sister's in college and we're really close. Last time she was home visiting, she told me about a secret club she and her friends had formed. Once a week, they eat all kinds of fattening food. They start with burgers, french fries, and milk shakes. Then, they get a dozen donuts. Later they split a pizza. After they've eaten all that food, they make themselves sick and get rid of it all. My sister was proud of the fact that she doesn't even have to stick her finger down her throat to vomit; she can just make herself do it. I was worried, but she says I'm being silly. She insists she only does it once a week and can stop any time she wants. Should I tell my parents?

Answer: The easy answer is yes, tell your parents. You're right to be worried about your sister, because she is abusing her body every week. Her once-a-week ritual can easily become a full-blown, uncontrollable eating disorder. If you're worried about betraying your sister's confidence, doing the right thing can be extremely hard. If you just can't do it, you should give your sister some information on how bingeing and purging is hurting her body and ask her to stop doing it.

Check the Hotlines and Help Sites section at the end of this book to find out how to get help.

TREATING BULIMIA

Experts who treat bulimia usually focus on three areas in their attempt to end the dangerous binge and purge cycle: **nutritional rehabilitation, psychosocial intervention,** and medication management.

People who suffer from bulimia often skip meals and later feel so hungry and out of control that they binge. Nutritional rehabilitation focuses on establishing a regular eating pattern. Research shows that those who eat regular meals are less likely to experience hunger and therefore feel less deprived. In turn, they are less likely to have as many binges.

Psychosocial intervention is an attempt to work through the emotional problems that contribute to bulimia through individual or group **psychotherapy.** The focus is on identifying the underlying emotional problems, improving **self-esteem,** and changing attitudes about food, weight, and appearance.

In some cases, physicians treat bulimia with **psychopharmacological drugs,** or drugs that affect the brain and central nervous system. If psychotherapy has not been completely successful, they may prescribe an **antidepressant** to control depression and **anxiety**—feelings of unease and fear. Once the bulimia is under control, the medication may help prevent **relapses.**

The possibility of a relapse is an important concern. Several studies cited by Healthy People 2010 show that after going into **remission** (having no binge-and-purge episodes for at least four weeks), about 25 percent have a relapse in less than three months. After nine months, 49 percent remained in remission. After four years with no symptoms of bulimia, the risk of relapse seems to decline.

TEENS SPEAK

How My Bulimia Began

I was skinny as a little girl. I loved picking out new clothes with my mom or dad and I especially loved the attention I got from my family and their friends who thought I was "just so cute."

I guess I was around 13 years old when I started getting a little pudgy. When my clothes got tight, my mom said I was just growing and took me out for more clothes. When I tried them on, I got upset because my stomach poked out a little. I wanted to look like my mother, with her flat stomach and thin legs. She did the best she could by helping me find styles that hid my stomach.

When summer rolled around and I put on a bathing suit, all I could think about was how great the water would feel. But when I took my cover-up off, my father teased me about my "beer belly." He hadn't been on the shopping trips and didn't know I was more than a little sensitive about the subject. He also wasn't about to enter high school and be confronted by skinny, popular girls.

I tried not to worry about my body, and my mother told me it was normal to go through a "chubby stage." But I did worry and worry. When I wasn't worrying, I was watching TV shows and movies about high school kids and fantasizing about what it would be like to live their lives. Who wouldn't want to be thin, cute, and popular?

Then, one day at the pool I was talking to a new girl, Brianna. After we had some ice cream, she told me she had to throw it up so she wouldn't get fat like her older sister. I couldn't believe what she had said. She took me to the bathroom and showed me how she made herself throw up. It really wasn't hard and I felt good afterward, I really did. A light bulb went off in my head, as I found the solution to my problems—I would be skinny by the time school started and I had a new best friend.

TAKING BULIMIA SERIOUSLY

Two fizzy tablets may make you feel better after eating a huge meal. Unfortunately, they can't alleviate the physical dangers of bingeing and purging or, more importantly, the emotional distress that underlies the behavior. Intentionally vomiting occasionally— only after you've really overeaten, for example—is not to be taken lightly and can easily turn into a true eating disorder. Bulimia is a serious health problem that should be treated as soon as it's discovered.

See also: Depression and Weight; Eating Disorders, Causes of; Eating Disorders, Symptoms and Diagnosis of; Media and Eating Disorders; Morbidity and Mortality; Nutrition and Nutritional Deficiencies; Treatment; Women and Eating Disorders

FURTHER READING

Costin, Carolyn. *The Eating Disorder Sourcebook: A Comprehensive Guide to the Causes, Treatments, and Prevention of Eating Disorders,* 3d ed. New York: McGraw/Hill, 2007.

Hall, Lindsey, and Leigh Cohn, M.A.T. *Bulimia: A Guide to Recovery.* Carlsbad, Calif.: Gurze Books, 1999. (Also available in Spanish as *Como entender y superar la bulimia*)

Keel, Pamela. *Eating Disorders.* New York: Chelsea House, 2006.

Normandi, Carol Emery, and Laurelee Roark. *Over It: A Teen's Guide to Getting Beyond Obsessions with Food and Weight.* Novato, Calif.: New World Library, 2001.

■ CALORIC INTAKE AND EXPENDITURES

Calories are the units of energy content in food. If you eat 3,500 extra calories without burning them off through exercise, you will gain a pound. For every 3,500 calories you burn off or remove from your normal food intake, you will lose a pound. Many Americans eat large portions and burn very few calories—a recipe for weight gain.

Health experts debate what makes people fat. Is fat okay as long as you avoid **carbohydrates**? Are cookies okay as long as they are non-fat? Different nutritionists say different things, but they do agree that 3,500 **calories** equals one pound.

CALORIES ARE NOT ALL BAD

Calories are used to measure how much energy various foods and drinks contain. You need energy to live, so calories are not a bad thing unless you take in more calories than your body needs. Once your body has used the calories it needs, the rest are turned into fat.

Your body receives four calories from every gram of **protein** or carbohydrate you eat and nine calories from every gram of fat. That's right, fat is responsible for twice as many calories as other nutrients. Most nutritionists recommend limiting calories from fat to 30 percent or less of total food intake.

Fact Or Fiction?

A hundred extra calories can't make a difference.

The Facts: The International Food Information Council Foundation (IFIC) claims that just 100 extra calories a day may be responsible for the increasing number of overweight people in the United States. Trimming just 100 calories a day could make a difference to your health. To trim those extra calories choose lower calorie foods, increase exercise, or try a combination of both.

The IFIC offers several suggestions for cutting 100 calories a day. For example, you could split a small bag of fries with a friend instead of eating the whole bag. Or you might replace a tablespoon of regular mayonnaise with one of fat-free mayonnaise or a teaspoon of mustard or ketchup. To burn about 100 calories, the IFIC recommends walking quickly for 22 minutes, cleaning the house for 25 minutes, or fast dancing for 16 minutes. To cut calories through a combination of exercise and food choices, eat 5 fewer potato chips and walk for 6 minutes or eat about a fourth cup less spaghetti with tomato sauce and walk for 11 minutes.

THE RIGHT NUMBER OF CALORIES

The number of calories you should be eating each day is different from the number of calories your mother or a baby brother should be eating. That's because the number of calories you need is based on your size, age, gender, and activity level. So, when you sit around the table at dinner with your family, it may be just fine that you are eating larger portions than your mother and that your baby brother is eating less than both of you. If you learn about your own nutritional needs, then you'll know whether you're eating the right amount of calories or not.

The U.S. Department of Agriculture (USDA) provides dietary guidelines every five years and has been making nutritional recommendations for more than 100 years. The 2005 guidelines recommend that teenage girls between the ages of 14 and 18 consume 1,800 to 2,400 calories a day, depending on their activity level, and that boys in the same age range aim for 2,200 to 3,200 calories a day.

Have you ever noticed the "Nutrition Facts" labels on packaged foods? Have you wondered who figured out how many calories a product has and how they did it? Scientists measure the calories in a food by burning it. The scientific name for the process is direct calorimetry and the instrument they use is called a **bomb calorimeter**—basically an insulated box with an oxygen-rich chamber surrounded by water. Food samples are placed in the box and then burned. The calorie count is equal to the increase in the temperature of the water around the box. In other words, if the temperature of the water increases by 10 degrees centigrade, the food has 10 calories.

Q & A

Question: How do I know what guidelines to follow?

Answer: With all the debate over nutrition, it is easy to become confused, but several places offer reliable information. The American Dietetic Association (ADA), the National Academy of Sciences (NAS), the USDA, and the Surgeon General's Office are all reputable sources. If you are doing research on the Web, keep in mind that as more and more research is done, scientists may change their recommendations. Always check the date of any report to make sure you are looking at the most up-to-date information.

CALORIES IN

Figuring out how many calories are in the foods you eat takes just a little effort. You can check the labels on foods you buy at the grocery store. Many cookbooks and magazines include nutrition information at the end of every recipe. Fast food and other restaurants may post the number of calories in various dishes or provide them on request. Dozens of books and Web sites are also devoted to counting calories.

Knowing about calories can help you make good nutritional choices. For example, an average slice of cheesecake contains 300 calories and an average slice of devil's food cake around 165. A cup of whole milk has 150 calories and a cup of skim milk, 86. An ounce of cheddar cheese contains 114 calories and an ounce of feta cheese, 75. If you choose to eat four ounces of dark meat chicken, you're eating 40 more calories than if you had chosen four ounces of white meat. A whole potato contains 114 calories—until you fry it! A small order of fries has about 200 calories and a large order more than 500! Choosing a slice of thin-crust cheese pizza instead of pan pizza saves about 90 calories. Choose diet soda (or better yet, water) instead of 8 ounces of regular soda and you save 100 calories. It's all about choices.

CALORIES OUT

Figuring out how many calories you work off when you exercise is easy. Books and Web sites offer information and so do many of the exercise machines at the gym. The amount of calories you burn depends on your weight as well as the exercise itself.

According to the calorie counter at the WebMD Health Web site, swimming is one of the best calorie burners. Surprisingly, you burn more calories with the breaststroke than the crawl. If you weigh 100 pounds, you can burn 147 calories in 20 minutes by swimming the breaststroke. If you weigh 150 pounds, you can burn 221 calories in 20 minutes. If you like to run, you can burn even more calories during that same 20 minutes. A 100-pound person running a seven-minute mile burns 207 calories in 20 minutes and a 150-pound person burns 311. If you run for 20 minutes at a more moderate pace (perhaps running an $11^1/_2$-minute mile), you will burn 123 calories if you weigh 100 pounds and 184 calories if you weigh 150 pounds.

Aerobic exercises like swimming and running, which raise your heart rate and make you breathe heavily, burn the most calories. But keep in mind that strengthening exercises that increase your muscle mass pay off, too, because the more muscular you are, the more calories you'll burn during aerobic exercise.

CALORIES AREN'T THE ENEMY

For many people who worry about their weight, calories are the enemy. Without calories, however, they would not have the energy to worry about them.

You can keep your body healthy by understanding how many calories your body needs. Then make sure that the calories you eat and the calories you burn through exercise add up to the right amount.

See also: Exercise; Fad Diets; Nutrition and Nutritional Deficiencies; Weight Control

■ DEPRESSION AND WEIGHT

Depression is a mental disorder characterized by feelings of sadness, despair, and discouragement, sometimes accompanied by weight problems. People who experience depression often have feelings of low **self-esteem**, guilt, and self-reproach. They may withdraw from relationships and show physical symptoms such as eating and sleep disturbances. Depression ranges from feeling blue to clinical depression—a mental state that requires professional intervention.

Which comes first—depression or a weight problem? Sometimes it is hard to say, but whether the issue is eating too much or too little, weight and depression are often linked. Problems may start with feeling bad about how your body looks. You're too fat, too skinny, too short, or too tall. You've got bad hair or the wrong color eyes or skin that's going through unsightly growing pains. Your body used to be okay, until it started changing too quickly or too slowly. The more self-conscious you feel, the more likely you are to succumb to peer pressure and risky behaviors.

Some people try alcohol, drugs, or sex to escape their own negative feelings or to feel more popular. Other people worry so much about their physical appearance that they feel worthless. They can't measure up to their own expectations, because they define themselves solely by how they think their body looks. This is the point at which depression can set in.

Experts have a hard time quantifying how many people suffer from depression, because it often goes undiagnosed. "The Numbers Count: Mental Disorders in America," published by the National Institute of Mental Health (NIMH), reports that data published in 2005 shows approximately 21 million adults have a mood disorder, which may be major depression, dysthymia, or bipolar disorder. Teens are also affected. The 2007 Youth Risk Behavior Surveillance study found that more than 28 percent of students surveyed reported that they avoided their usual activities because of ongoing feelings of sadness or hopelessness.

In assessing teenage depression, the 2007 Youth Risk Behavior Survey asked high school students whether they felt "so sad or hopeless almost every day for more than two weeks in a row that they stopped doing some usual activities." They also asked whether the students had seriously considered attempting suicide any time during the 12 months preceding the survey.

Mental health professionals categorize depression by degree or type. **Major depression** is the most severe depressive disorder. Those suffering from major depression exhibit several symptoms of depression and their condition significantly interferes with their ability to meet responsibilities and take part in or enjoy everyday activities. Some people experience major depression just once in their lives. About half of those who have experienced it once are likely to experience one or more additional episodes later in life.

Dysthymia is another depressive disorder. Although its symptoms are milder than those of a major depression, it is a chronic condition, which means that it lasts for a long time. Dysthymia can keep people from feeling good or doing things they want to do. Someone who suffers from dysthymia is likely to also experience a major depression.

Bipolar disorder is less common than the other two depressive disorders, affecting nearly 6 million adults, according to "The Numbers Count." Also known as manic-depressive disorder, bipolar disorder is characterized by large mood swings, with very high "ups" and very low "downs." The changes in mood are usually gradual but can also be sudden. Bipolar disorder can occur at any age but the median age of onset is 25.

Those who experience a manic episode (a high) may feel that they are on top of the world; everything seems bigger and brighter than before. They are full of ideas, the world is full of possibilities, and they are eager to share their exuberance and **euphoria** with others. While it sounds wonderful, it can actually progress to a state of **psychosis** characterized by **hallucinations, delusions,** or other major mental dysfunctions. At other times, mania is not euphoric at all. Some people become extremely irritable, distracted, aggressive, and abusive during a manic episode. Either way, the mania eventually goes away and depression begins.

Fact Or Fiction?

Depression is just a mood, and if you really want to you can snap out of it.

The Facts: Depression is much more than a bad mood. It is an illness that affects the mind, body, behavior, and mood. The good news is that 80 percent of people suffering from depression can get better with treatment, according to *Depression: What You Need To Know,* a publication issued by Mental Health America. Treatment may involve medication or psycho-therapy or both. But even with the help of a mental health professional, getting over depression is a gradual process.

RECOGNIZING SYMPTOMS

Like everyone, you experience bad moods, sadness, boredom, loneli-ness, or even vague feelings of just being "out of it." You have prob-ably said you were depressed. Are you just feeling blue or are you experiencing depression? Anyone who has a bad mood that lasts two weeks or more, feels great despair, isn't doing well in school or enjoy-ing time with friends, or has experienced a change in sleeping and eating habits should seek help. This is particularly true for those who have had thoughts about **suicide.**

The symptoms of depression aren't always the same. Some people become withdrawn and quiet while others are angry and act in ways that are meant to attract attention. The shy person whose clothing fades into the background and the outgoing person with purple hair may look and act differently, but both could be suffering from the same basic disorder.

DID YOU KNOW?

High School Students and Depression

	Felt sad or hopeless	Seriously considered attempting suicide	Made a suicide plan	Attempted suicide	Suicide attempts required medical attention
Female	35.8%	18.7%	13.4%	9.3%	2.4%
Male	21.2%	10.3%	9.2%	4.6%	1.5%

Source: Youth Risk Behavior Survey, 2007.

Depression can be caused by many outside factors—the stress of a new stage in life, a breakup, a traumatic event, or a death in the family. Depression may also be caused by a chemical imbalance in the brain. You have chemical messengers in your brain called **neurotransmitters** that make you feel happy, satisfied, and energized. When that message system goes awry, depression can be the result.

Those experiencing depression can have one symptom or many. The symptoms can be more or less severe and they may change over time. The NIMH lists the following as symptoms of depression:

- persistent sad, anxious or "empty" mood;
- feelings of hopelessness or pessimism;
- feelings of guilt, worthlessness, and helplessness;
- loss of interest or pleasure in hobbies and activities that were once enjoyed;
- decreased energy, fatigue, and being "slowed down";
- difficulty concentrating, remembering, and making decisions;
- insomnia, early-morning awakening, or oversleeping;
- appetite and/or weight loss, or overeating and weight gain;
- thoughts of death or suicide or suicide attempts;
- restlessness and irritability; and
- persistent physical symptoms that do not respond to treatment, such as headaches, digestive disorders, and chronic pain.

Q & A

Question: Is depression genetic?

Answer: According to a 2007 publication on depression issued by the National Institute of Mental Health, current research suggests that a vulnerability to depression may be genetic. That is, if a family member or several generations of family members have experienced clinical depression, you may also be at risk—that does not mean you will experience depression but that you are more vulnerable to it. Furthermore, many people who experience depression do not have a family history of depression. So family history seems to be just one of many factors that can play into depression.

WEIGHT LOSS

Weight loss is a common symptom of depression. People who are depressed often lose interest in things that are normally pleasurable to them, and eating can be one of those things. They may lack the energy to prepare or buy food. They may also avoid social situations, which almost always involve food. As they become thinner and their clothes become baggy, they may not care because they have lost interest in their physical appearance.

People who are actively trying to lose weight may think a little depression would be welcome if the weight came off more easily. Depression, however, is not something to wish for. In fact, people who are trying to lose weight should be especially wary of depression. If you lose weight and then gain it back, your self-esteem goes up and down, too, and the result can be depression.

TEENS SPEAK

Depressed over Heather

Heather was my first serious girlfriend. I'd liked other girls before, but not the way I liked Heather. In fact, after we'd been going out for a year, I told her I loved her—and meant it. Now that I look back on it, the day I told Heather I loved her was the beginning of the end. You can probably guess that she didn't say "I love you" back. It took about two weeks before she said the last thing any guy in love wants to hear—"we need to talk." With college just a few months away, Heather didn't want a hometown boyfriend dragging her down.

I told her I understood, but I was crushed. I tried to study for final exams but had serious concentration problems. I spent hours with my books open, but the words seemed to float off the page. At night, I had trouble falling asleep and then trouble staying asleep. When I did sleep, I had some pretty awful nightmares.

I was hardly eating anything. In the mornings, after a fitful night's sleep, I would have a hard time getting up, so I would run out of the house without breakfast. At school, I avoided the cafeteria because I'd see Heather there. At dinner, I just couldn't make the food go down. My parents became concerned. They tried to talk to me about Heather and told me stories about how they got dumped and how they got over it. They tried jokes, bribes, threats, and punishments, but none of it mattered to me. I just didn't feel happy anymore and I just wanted to be left alone. I was going through the motions at school and that was about it.

Then, one day my uncle came over. I answered the door, said hello, and then went back to my room. As I walked away, I heard him talking to my mom. He didn't understand why I wasn't happy to see him and he couldn't believe how much weight I'd lost. My mom told him it was "about a girl" and even though she was worried, she was sure I'd be back to normal as soon as school was out. My uncle reminded her that their mother used to react the same way. Anything stressful or disappointing would totally debilitate her for weeks. He suggested I see a psychologist and be screened for depression. It turned out to be a life-saving suggestion.

WEIGHT GAIN

One of the odd things about depression is that it may lead some people to lose weight and others to gain weight. In fact, weight gain can be both a cause and an effect of depression.

Depression may cause people to gain weight, because it can slow them down. The more time they spend sleeping and avoiding activity and exercise, the more likely that their **metabolism** will slow and they will feel tired all the time.

Overeating or eating without concern for nutrition may also be the result of negative, pessimistic feelings. People think, "Who cares if I get fat?" At that point, a vicious cycle begins. As they gain weight their self-esteem plummets, their depression worsens, and their weight goes higher and higher.

Q & A

Question: Can antidepressants make me gain weight?

Answer: Yes. Weight gain is listed as a side effect of a number of psychopharmacological drugs used to treat depression and bipolar disorder. That's because many of these medications are designed to affect the body's level of a neurotransmitter called serotonin. Serotonin doesn't just affect mood; it can also affect appetite and metabolism. However, the weight gain seems to be affected by one's genes.

EATING PATTERNS

Those who suffer from bulimia and depression will often **binge** because they are depressed and then after purging, become depressed again. **Compulsive** eaters also use food to overcome depression. This use of food becomes an **addiction** and results in a dangerous cycle— bingeing leads to depression, which leads to more bingeing, and on and on.

Eating a balanced diet, on the other hand, may help ward off depression. Some researchers feel that if you suffer from depression, eating the recommended amount (six to 11 servings) of **carbohydrates** may make you feel better, because carbohydrates affect how much serotonin your body produces, and **serotonin** affects mood, appetite, and metabolism. However, studies also suggest that the amino acid tryptophan is necessary in producing serotonin, which would require eating protein. The *American Dietetic Association Complete Food and Nutrition Guide* reports that a deficiency in Vitamin B_6 (pyridoxine)— which is found in chicken, fish, pork, liver, and kidney—can cause depression.

Some researchers believe that low levels of **Omega-3 fatty acids**, which are found in fish oils, may also be linked to depression. In May 2001, researchers at the University of Kuopio in Finland evaluated 1,767 men and women and found that regular fish consumption reduced the risk of depression and suicide. Their results were consistent with a Japanese study in which 265,000 subjects were followed for 17 years. Eating foods with Omega-3 fatty acids, such as salmon, sardines, and flaxseed, may help prevent depression.

Fact Or Fiction?

If you're feeling depressed, an alcoholic drink can improve your mood.

The Facts: Alcohol is a depressant. Although you may think it will make you feel better, it will actually deepen your depression.

THE WEIGHT OF DEPRESSION

Depression affects people in different ways. One person suffering from depression may turn to food for comfort. Another may forget to eat or feel unable to eat during a bout with depression. Either way, depression is likely to affect one's body weight. Researchers are hopeful that new studies may improve the diagnosis and treatment of this serious and all too common mental illness.

See also: Eating Disorders, Causes of; Eating Disorders, Symptoms and Diagnosis of; Morbidity and Mortality; Stress and Eating Habits

FURTHER READING

Clarke, Julie M., and Ann Kirby-Payne. *Understanding Weight and Depression.* New York: Rosen Publishing Group, 2000.

Denkmire, Heather. *The Truth About Fear and Depression.* New York: Facts On File, 2005.

National Institute of Mental Health. "Depression in Children and Adolescents: A Fact Sheet for Physicians." September 2002.

——. "The Numbers Count: Mental Disorders in America." URL: http://www.nimh.nih.gov/health/publications/the-numbers-count-mental-disorders-in-america.shtml/#Eating. Updated May 28, 2008.

■ DIET PILLS

Medications and supplements intended to help people lose weight by suppressing the appetite. There are a wide variety on the market, many of which have addictive qualities and serious side effects.

Losing weight through diet and exercise is hard work. So the thought of taking a pill that will melt the fat away may be as tempting as chocolate candy or french fries or whatever food is your dieting downfall.

Some people need to lose weight in order to be healthy. They may mistakenly turn to diet pills because they are overwhelmed or frustrated by the effort that healthy dieting requires. Others, including those with anorexia or bulimia who are already punishing their bodies in a multitude of ways, may also be attracted to diet pills.

People who hope that a pill will solve their weight problem have a variety of prescription and **over-the-counter** medications to choose from. They may also be attracted to products labeled as dietary, nutritional or herbal **supplements**—different names for the same things. These supplements are not tested and regulated the way prescription and over-the-counter medications are, because they do not require approval by the Food and Drug Administration (FDA). The FDA can remove unsafe supplements from the market; an herbal supplement known as ephedra has been banned from the marketplace by the FDA since April 2004.

Those concerned about safety may feel reassured by the fact that the FDA reviews all medications before they are allowed on the market. Yet, even then, there's still no guarantee that the medication is completely safe. In the 1990s, the FDA recalled several diet drugs that were previously approved.

Although diet pills can be part of a strategy that includes cutting **calories**, exercising, and therapy, they also can be deadly. Although many different diet pills are on the market, they tend to fall into one of two categories—those that no one should take because they cause more harm than good and those that should be taken only under the supervision of a physician.

PRESCRIPTION OBESITY DRUGS

In 1999 the FDA approved the first in a new class of obesity drugs known as **lipase inhibitors**. Called Xenical, the drug works in the intestines, blocking the amount of **fat** the body absorbs by as much as 30 percent. Undigested fat is then eliminated during bowel movements. When the body absorbs less fat, it retains fewer calories. For the seriously obese who are not able to lose weight through diet and exercise alone, Xenical is a promising treatment. However, like all diet drugs, it can have serious side effects. According to the FDA, Xenical's main side effects include "cramping, diarrhea, flatulence, intestinal discomfort, and leakage of oily stool."

Other prescription diet drugs suppress appetite by increasing brain chemicals. The FDA approved one such drug known as Meridia (sibutramine) in 1997 with this warning: "Because it may increase blood pressure and heart rate, Meridia should not be used by people with uncontrolled **high blood pressure**, a history of heart disease, congestive heart failure, irregular heartbeat, or **stroke**. Other common side effects of Meridia include headache, dry mouth, constipation, and insomnia."

Many years ago, the FDA also approved Bontril (phendimetrazine tartrate), Desoxyn (methamphetamine), and Ionamin and Adipex-P (phentermine) for short-term use. The FDA warns that these are "'speed'-like drugs that should not be used by people with heart disease, high blood pressure, an overactive thyroid gland, or glaucoma." Side effects may include blurred vision, dizziness, dry mouth, sleeplessness, irritability, stomach upset, and constipation. These drugs generally don't help with weight loss for more than a few weeks, and they can be highly addictive.

Several obesity drugs—fenfluramine (Pondimin and others), exfenfluramine (Redux), and a combination of fenfluramine and phentermine (Fen-Phen)—received a lot of publicity in the 1990s. In 1997, the FDA recalled them, based on scientific evidence that they may cause heart valve problems.

OVER-THE-COUNTER DIET PILLS

In February 2007, the FDA approved GlaxoSmithKline's alli™. Alli, a reduced-strength version of Xenical, is the only FDA-approved over-the-counter weight-loss product. The drug is approved for adults 18 years and older and is designed to be part of an overall weight/loss plan that includes a healthy diet and exercise.

The FDA has banned a large number of over-the-counter diet products, because the ingredients are believed to be dangerous. Others have been removed from sale because manufacturers were unable to prove the claims they made about their products. In 1992, the FDA banned 111 ingredients—including amino acids, cellulose, and grapefruit extract—because companies failed to prove that these ingredients contribute to the kind of weight loss promised in their advertising.

Several products were recalled because they contain guar gum. Guar gum is supposed to work by swelling the stomach so that a person feels full. Unfortunately it can also cause dangerous blockages in the stomach and throat. Cal-Ban 3000, Cal-Lite 1000, Cal-Trim 5000, Perma Slim, Bodi Trim, Dictol 7 Plus, Medi Thin, Nature's Way, and East Indian Guar Gum were all banned because they contain this ingredient.

Phenylpropanolamine is an active ingredient used until recently in both over-the-counter diet pills and nasal decongestants. In 2000, the FDA issued a public health advisory warning people to stop taking drugs that contain phenylpropanolamine. The department also asked manufacturers of diet pills that contain the ingredient to reformulate their products.

Phenylpropanolamine is linked to an increased risk of hemorrhagic stroke (bleeding in the brain). Dexatrim and Acutrim are some of the brand-name diet aids that used to contain phenylpropanolamine.

In 2003, ephedra became the first dietary supplement to be banned by the FDA. The controversial diet aid, which claimed to increase weight loss and improve athletic performance, was linked to 16,000 adverse reactions, including strokes, heart attacks, and irregular heart-beats. The FDA also attributed 92 deaths to the supplement, including that of a 23-year-old pitcher for the Baltimore Orioles. Even before the FDA took action, three states—Illinois, New York, and California—had passed laws banning ephedra. The National Football League, college sports teams, and the International Olympic Committee all prohibit athletes from using the supplement.

In 2003, a RAND Corporation study commissioned by the National Institutes of Health supported these actions and earlier studies that indicated ephedra poses significant health risks (particularly to the nervous system and heart), while showing only limited health benefits. Known side effects of ephedra include nervousness, **anxiety**, high blood pressure, insomnia, dizziness, lightheadedness, and heart palpitations.

Over-the-counter drugs have "Drug Facts" labels similar to the "Nutrition Facts" labels on food packaging. These labels make it easy to identify side effects associated with the medication, active ingredients, proper dosage, and FDA warnings about the medication. Supplements also contain labels. Although these labels include a list of ingredients, they do not provide as much information as is found on drug labels. Some list warnings and side effects; others do not. Often consumers have to read the very small print to learn more about the product.

Because the FDA doesn't maintain information on supplements the way it does on drugs, it recommends that consumers contact the manufacturer directly if they want more information about a supplement. The manufacturer's name and address are on the label. Consumers can also search the Internet for news stories and other information on specific supplements. It's always a good idea to check the date the information was posted and make sure the Web site is maintained by a legitimate, knowledgeable organization.

Fact Or Fiction?

As long as I stick to "all-natural" diet products, I'll be safe.

The Facts: Many substances found in nature are toxic, so claims that a dietary supplement is "natural" or "herbal" should not fool you into assuming it is safe. In fact, you should be more cautious when considering the use of dietary supplements because the FDA does not review them. Like other pharmaceutical products, ingredients found in supplements may interact negatively with drugs or be dangerous to people with certain medical conditions.

DIET PILL OF THE FUTURE

With all the advances in medicine, it may be hard to believe that scientists have not yet come up with a pharmaceutical solution to weight loss—one that allows you to eat whatever you want without worrying about becoming fat. But it hasn't happened yet.

See also: Caloric Intake and Expenditures; Fad Diets; Laxative Abuse; Weight Control

FURTHER READING

Clayton, Lawrence. *Diet Pill Drug Dangers*. Berkeley Heights, N.J.: Enslow Publishing, 2001.
Williams, Karen. *Diet Drugs*. New York: Rosen Publishing, 2007.

■ DIETING

See: Caloric Intake and Expenditures; Diet Pills; Fad Diets

■ EATING DISORDERS, CAUSES OF

Psychological disorders characterized by a compulsive obsession with food or weight. Anorexia and bulimia are eating disorders.

Who—or what—is to blame for an eating disorder? When looking at causes, many factors are involved. Mental health, peer pressure, family issues, genetics, society, and the media can all play a role.

PSYCHOLOGICAL DIFFICULTIES

Depression, loneliness, poor self-esteem, substance abuse, feelings of inadequacy, anger, and **anxiety** are common among people who develop eating disorders. In December 2004, the American Psychiatric Association published a study conducted by a research team that included noted eating disorder experts Walter H. Kaye and Cynthia M. Bulik. The researchers were looking at how often anxiety disorders occurred along with anorexia or bulimia and found that about two-thirds of the eating disorder patients they studied had an anxiety disorder. Most patients had developed the anxiety disorder while they were children, before developing their eating disorder. The numbers were the same regardless of whether the patients had anorexia, bulimia, or both.

In March 2008, researchers at University of Virginia reported that girls with attention-deficit/hyperactivity disorder (ADHD) may have a "substantially greater risk" of developing symptoms of bulimia. Lead researcher Amori Mikami said that girls with ADHD are impulsive, and that may make it harder for them to maintain healthy eating habits. Her study included more than 220 girls in the San Francisco Bay area, evaluated twice, once between the ages of six and 12 and again five years later.

Those who are praised or ridiculed for their weight or sexual development are also at greater risk of having an eating disorder, according to Anorexia Nervosa and Related Eating Disorders, Inc. (ANRED). So are victims of sexual or physical abuse.

An eating disorder may be an attempt to create an identity that equates thinness with popularity and success. Later, the eating disorder may begin to define one's identity, making it more difficult to let go. If you aren't bulimic anymore, who are you? What will make you different, or special, compared to others?

Some people have strong feelings of anger and no outlet or ability for expressing that anger in a healthy way. The anger becomes a self-inflicted wound, in the form of an eating disorder.

DEFICIENT SOCIAL SKILLS

In American society, eating is a social event. Every holiday has its own special foods. Sociologists and psychologists claim that families that make a habit of eating dinner together tend to be closer. People also may eat to be polite or please someone, like a grandmother who baked all day in preparation for a visit.

It's no wonder, given the connection between food and social situations, that poor social skills and eating disorders are often connected. Not everyone with an eating disorder has social problems, but many do. As they grow older, some people find the need to develop new social skills difficult, frightening, and stressful. Often the way they handle a social situation may be colored by how they feel about the way they look.

An eating disorder is often used as a substitute for acceptable social behavior. Those who are unsure of their social skills may focus their energy on food instead of interacting with friends. They may eat for comfort and company, or they may compulsively diet or **binge** and purge in a misguided effort to be thin and popular.

As an eating disorder develops, social skills may deteriorate. People with eating disorders often lie, avoid social situations that involve food (and most social situations do), or withdraw from friends and others to hide what they're doing.

FAMILY INFLUENCES

Eating disorders are often caused by a troubled relationship within the family. For example, an eating disorder may be a call for attention by someone who is part of a family that doesn't communicate well.

Another factor may be the amount of emotional support a child receives from his or her parents. The way parents nurture their children impacts the youngsters' ability to care for themselves. Those who have not received adequate nurturing may think they don't deserve to be looked after, and deprive themselves of food as a result. Alternatively, they may turn to food for comfort.

Even loving and nurturing families may inadvertently send signals that lead to an eating disorder—perhaps by overemphasizing thinness and exercise or having overly high expectations. Young people who feel smothered by overprotective parents may use eating and exercising as a means of exhibiting independence and self-control.

Some girls develop anorexia because they are afraid to separate from their parents, especially their mothers. In effect, they halt their sexual development as a way to avoid leaving childhood.

Those with mothers who have experienced an eating disorder may be at a higher risk of developing an eating disorder than those whose parents don't have prominent food issues. The reason? A mother with an eating disorder is likely to approach food and nutrition differently. Genetic factors, discussed below, can affect the likelihood of developing an eating disorder as well.

Other family relationships also can play a role in causing an eating disorder. Sibling rivalry or the desire to be like an older sibling may increase the risk of an eating disorder. Later, a difficult relationship with a spouse may prove to be as dangerous as a troubled relationship with a parent.

GENETIC CAUSES

Many researchers are studying how genetic factors may contribute to the development of eating disorders. University of North Carolina at Chapel Hill researcher Cynthia M. Bulik, Ph.D., studied more than 30,000 Swedish twins and concluded in 2006 that 56 percent of anorexia cases were genetically linked. In 2007, researchers who looked at another twin study, the Minnesota Twin Family Study, found that genetic effects were especially prevalent in girls between the ages of 14 and 18. In 2002, *Eating Disorders Review* reported that anyone with a mother or sister who suffers from an eating disorder is 12 times more likely to develop anorexia and four times more likely to develop bulimia. In March 2003, the *New England Journal of Medicine* published a study done by researchers in Switzerland, Germany, and the United States. It suggests that heredity is an important factor in the development of obesity and binge eating for some, but not all, people.

In March 2002, the *American Journal of Psychiatry* published a study conducted by researchers from the University of California, Los Angeles, and Western Psychiatric Institute in Pittsburgh which included nearly 2,000 sisters or mothers of 504 young adult women with anorexia or bulimia. They found that relatives of women with anorexia were 11 times more likely to have anorexia and relatives of women with bulimia had an almost four times greater risk for bulimia.

The study also found a connection between the two eating disorders. Relatives of women with bulimia had a 12 times higher risk for anorexia and relatives of women with anorexia were 3.5 times more likely to develop bulimia, when compared with people who had no family history of eating disorders.

Some studies have focused on whether **neurochemistry** may play a role in some eating disorders. **Serotonin** and **neuroepinephrine** are **neurotransmitters** that give you a sense of physical and emotional fulfillment. Serotonin, in particular, sends the message that you feel full and have had enough to eat. Researchers have found that acutely ill patients suffering from anorexia and bulimia have significantly lower levels of serotonin and neuroepinephrine. The same neurotransmitters also function abnormally in people with depression, which is also often linked to eating disorders.

People with eating disorders tend to have higher than normal levels of the hormones vasopressin and cortisol. Both are released in response to stress. Levels of neuropeptide and peptide are also elevated in people with eating disorders. These substances have been shown to stimulate eating behavior in laboratory animals.

Scientists working with laboratory animals have identified yet another hormone known as cholecystokinin (CCK). They believe that it makes laboratory animals feel so full that they stop eating. People with bulimia tend to have low CCK levels.

SOCIAL INFLUENCES

In the United States, thin is an important part of the definition of the word *beauty*. Many believe that the fact that society glorifies thinness and encourages a quest for the "perfect body" may contribute to eating disorders. Society also tends to recognize, praise, and reward individuals based solely on their physical appearance. For example, do you remember the story of Cinderella? She and the prince fall in love at first sight. The very phrase *love at first sight* shows what a strong role physical appearance plays in definitions of beauty. More evidence can be found in models—men and women who use their appearance to sell products. In fact, the power of beauty can be seen throughout the business world. Many claim that tall, thin people are more likely to reach higher levels on the corporate ladder than people who are short and overweight.

For many young girls and women, a focus on appearance can increase the risk of an eating disorder. For example, the desire to look good for a boyfriend or girlfriend can turn into a dangerous obsession. Even membership in a social club, sorority, cheerleading squad, dance group, or "the popular crowd" (or the desire to belong) may encourage unhealthy eating habits. When you lose a little weight, through healthy or unhealthy means, and everyone at school tells you how great you look, the well-intentioned compliments may create a need for more compliments. That praise can be gained only through more and more dieting.

MEDIA EXPECTATIONS

The female images you see in the movies, in magazines, and on TV are overwhelmingly thin. The male images are overwhelmingly strong and virile. Is it any wonder, then, that so many women weaken themselves through diet while men try to strengthen themselves through exercise? (Not that there aren't plenty of women who exercise for strength and men who diet to become thin, but the majority is the other way around.)

Many sociologists blame super-thin supermodels and skinny actresses for hang-ups about weight. They point out that most fashion models are thinner than 98 percent of American women. The average American woman is 5'4" tall and weighs 140 pounds. The average model is 5'11" and weighs 117 pounds. These statistics come from a 1996 study by Professor Linda Smolak of Kenyon College. She and others use the **body mass index (BMI)** to make comparisons.

The powerful influence the media has on society has been documented in various studies. TV is especially influential. In 1999, for example, Anne Becker, a professor at Harvard Medical School, published a study describing Fiji, a small island in the Pacific, before and after the arrival of television. In 1995, before television came to the island, Fijians thought that the ideal body was round, plump, and soft. After three years of watching American TV programs, including shows like *Melrose Place* and *Beverly Hills 90210*, teenage girls in Fiji showed serious signs of eating disorders.

The Harvard study also found that Fijian females who watched TV three or more nights per week were 50 percent more likely to feel "too big" or "too fat" than people who watched less TV. About two-thirds of the TV-watching teens reported dieting in the previous month, and 15 percent said they had vomited to control their weight.

PHYSICAL CONDITIONS

Puberty is a time when teens become more conscious of their bodies. Girls who experience earlier sexual development than their peers may be more at risk of developing an eating disorder. As their bodies change shape, they may encounter several new feelings—fear at the prospect of leaving childhood, the discomfort of looking different from everyone else, and a lack of control as their bodies undergo

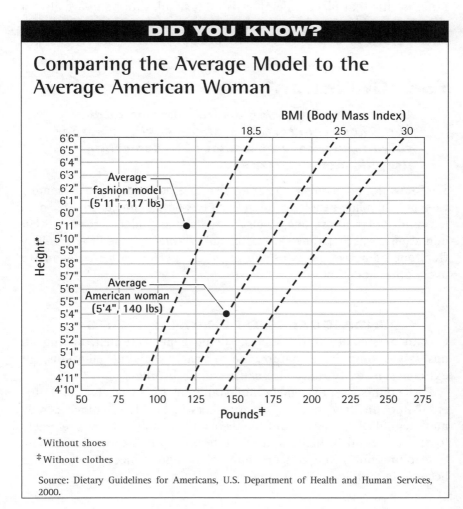

DID YOU KNOW?

Comparing the Average Model to the Average American Woman

*Without shoes

‡Without clothes

Source: Dietary Guidelines for Americans, U.S. Department of Health and Human Services, 2000.

changes. For these girls, dieting, bingeing, and purging can be an attempt to turn back the clock or exert control over their bodies.

Another physical condition that may contribute to an eating disorder is **diabetes**. People who are diabetic have to be very careful about what they eat. Unfortunately, some may become obsessive. In an effort to be health conscious, they actually do their bodies harm. The American Academy of Family Physicians reports that up to one-third of girls with type 1 diabetes are prone to eating disorders and are at high risk of developing serious health problems.

Male and female athletes who participate in ballet, gymnastics, and other events that place an emphasis on a small, thin body are also at risk. These athletes may go to extreme measures to lose weight in an attempt to be at what they consider peak physical form.

Fact Or Fiction?

Anyone with an eating disorder has an addiction. Those who recover from an eating disorder will probably become addicted to something else, like alcohol or drugs.

The Facts: Not all people with eating disorders have addictive personalities, but for some people an addictive personality can contribute to an eating disorder. These people also may have a tendency toward other addictions, whether they recover or not. However, a healthy recovery from one addictive behavior can provide a person with the means to avoid other addictions.

INDIVIDUAL AND PERSONAL TRAITS

Certain personality traits—such as being a **perfectionist**, having an **obsessive–compulsive** nature, not openly showing emotions, or extreme sensitivity—may also cause eating disorders.

Perfectionists set extremely high standards for themselves and others. Although they may appear to others to be high achievers, they may regard their accomplishments as inadequate. They are likely to see the world in black and white terms. Thin is good. Fat is bad. Controlling one's weight is one more challenge to meet. The behavior becomes an addiction.

Q & A

Question: Does the fact that I'm a teenager make me more likely to get an eating disorder?

Answer: Although anyone at any age can develop an eating disorder, the National Women's Health Resource Center reports that more than 90 percent of people diagnosed with anorexia and bulimia are women and that eating problems usually develop between the ages of 12 and 25. Young women may be susceptible to eating disorder because of the many physical and emotional changes they experience during adolescence, their vulnerability to peer pressure, and an extreme need to measure up to others. In fact, most adolescent girls are more afraid of gaining weight than getting cancer, confronting nuclear war, or losing their parents, according to a report by Rader Programs, a respected treatment center.

HISTORY OF EATING DISORDERS

Although modern society and the all-pervasive media are often blamed for eating disorders (and indeed have increased how often they occur), the problem has a long history.

In 1686, a physician in Europe documented what may be the earliest known case of anorexia. He described his 20-year-old female patient as "a skeleton only clad with skin" and made a clear distinction between her illness and a common disease of the time—tuberculosis.

Until recently, eating disorders were generally assumed to affect mainly young, white females. However, as awareness has grown and diagnosis has improved, researchers have learned that eating disorders know no boundaries. They affect all ethnicities, all ages, and both genders.

FROM CAUSE TO PREVENTION

Old, young, male, female, rich, poor—no one is immune from eating disorders. A variety of influences and personality traits may be at the root of an eating disorder. Recognizing potential causes is the first step in preventing an occurrence.

See also: Anorexia; Bulimia; Depression and Weight; Eating Disorders in Men and Boys; Media and Eating Disorders; Morbidity and Mortality; Peer Pressure; Self-Image; Women and Eating Disorders

FURTHER READING

Brumberg, Joan Jacobs. *Fasting Girls: The History of Anorexia Nervosa.* New York: Vintage Books, 2000.

Kirkpatrick, Jim, and Paul Caldwell. *Eating Disorders, Everything You Need to Know.* Buffalo, N.Y.: Firefly Books, 2001.

National Women's Health Resource Center. "Eating Disorders," National Women's Health Resource Center. URL: http://www. healthywomen.org/healthtopics/eatingdisorders. Updated March 8, 2007.

Zerbe, Kathryn J. *The Body Betrayed: A Deeper Understanding of Women, Eating Disorders and Treatment,* 1993. American Psychiatric Press, Inc., 1995. (Softcover edition, Carlsbad, Calif.: Gurze Books).

■ EATING DISORDERS, SYMPTOMS AND DIAGNOSIS OF

Psychological disorders characterized by a compulsive obsession with food or weight, eating disorders are considered diseases, because they have predictable symptoms and outcomes. If you recognize the signs in someone you know, don't keep your concern to yourself. The longer an eating disorder continues, the harder it is to recover, both emotionally and physically.

People with eating disorders generally try to hide their condition. They spend much of their time thinking and planning what to eat or not to eat and how to keep their secret from others. People with anorexia, who literally starve themselves, often try to look as if they have eaten more than they have. Some wear baggy clothes or even put weights in their pockets before being weighed at the doctor's office. People who **binge** are likely to eat normally in public and then find ways to eat huge quantities of food very quickly in private. Those who attempt to get rid of unwanted **calories** by purging (usu-ally vomiting) often look for out-of-the-way bathrooms where no one can hear what they're doing. Eventually, despite the deception, signs of an eating disorder become evident.

PHYSICAL SIGNS

Some signs of an eating disorder are things everyone suffers from occasionally—fatigue, dizziness, and stomachaches. Others, like dental problems and dramatic weight losses, are not common.

Therefore these signs of an eating disorder may be particularly telling.

Anorexia

One of the most conspicuous physical symptoms of anorexia is weight loss or, in the case of children and teenagers who are still growing, the absence of normal weight gain. Clinicians consider someone anorexic if his or her weight is 15 percent below the recommended body weight for height and age.

Despite their appearance, people with anorexia don't think they look thin (or at least not thin enough). They may feel bloated or full after eating just a small amount. They catch cold easily. The hair on their head becomes thinner, and very fine hair grows on their face and arms. They are often tired and have difficulty concentrating. Girls who have reached puberty usually stop menstruating or their periods become irregular.

Other physical signs are less obvious. People with anorexia have **low blood pressure** and may feel dizzy or faint easily. They may be depressed, anxious, or have trouble sleeping. They may have kidney or heart problems. Some experience stomach pain, heartburn and constipation, especially if they use laxatives. Those who induce vomiting are likely to have dental problems, because the acid from the vomit wears away tooth enamel.

Q & A

Question: My friend has lost a lot of weight lately. I asked her if she thought she might be anorexic and she said absolutely not. In fact, she said she had set up a doctor's appointment, because she was concerned about the weight loss. Is she just trying to hide an eating disorder?

Answer: The fact that your friend is concerned about her weight loss could mean that it is caused by a physical problem. Typically, people with anorexia deny their thinness, while people who are experiencing some other problem may be concerned about the loss of weight.

Bulimia

If someone is at either end of the weight scale—anorexic or obese— it is relatively easy to see he or she isn't leading a healthy life.

People suffering from bulimia are not as easy to detect. They are often able to maintain their weight. Despite their appearance, they may be so deficient in nutrients that they are actually starving their body—depriving themselves of what they need to grow or stay healthy.

Most of the physical problems associated with bulimia are due to purging. Vomiting brings up stomach acid, which can cause serious tooth decay and make salivary glands swell, giving the appearance of "chipmunk cheeks." The vomiting can also result in a dangerous loss of potassium. Purging may also lead to **dehydration**.

Like anorexia, bulimia places considerable stress on the organs of the body. Damage to the stomach and kidneys may result in constant stomach pain. Girls may also stop menstruating. Both males and females may experience a sharp drop in their potassium level, which may result in serious heart problems. People with bulimia also may be depressed, anxious, and have trouble sleeping.

Binge-eating disorder

People with a binge-eating disorder often feel compelled to eat abnormally large amounts of food in a short period of time. Unlike those with bulimia, they don't purge later. Yet they have many of the same physical symptoms as people who suffer from bulimia. The binges can cause painful tears in the stomach and sometimes bleeding. In rare cases, binge-eating may lead to a fatal stomach rupture. If someone with the disorder becomes obese, **diabetes**, **high blood pressure**, heart attack, and **stroke** are also possible. Half of those with a binge-eating disorder are **overweight**, so weight gain is yet another physical symptom.

BEHAVIORAL PATTERNS

What is "normal" behavior? Experts agree that it is not always easy to know. The teenage years are difficult, but people at every age wrestle with issues of identity, transitions in their lives, and setbacks. Knowing whether a behavior is an indicator of an eating disorder or just a sign that someone is going through a rough patch can be difficult. The important thing is not to brush off the feeling that something isn't quite right. If you recognize signs of an eating disorder in someone you know, talk to that person about those signs instead of ignoring them.

Anorexia

People with anorexia often have unusual eating habits. They may skip meals, declare certain foods off limits, refuse to eat meals with other people, eat very little, or become very strict about measuring portions. The fact that they are not eating doesn't mean they're avoiding food. On the contrary, they may show an intense interest in cooking, reading recipes, and watching cooking shows on TV. They may get vicarious enjoyment from cooking for others and watching them eat.

Those who have anorexia tend to weigh themselves often. Because the scale never shows a weight they consider too low, they also tend to exercise compulsively, vomit, or use laxatives, **diuretics**, and enemas to lose more weight.

Bulimia

People with bulimia are afraid of gaining weight. They will often skip meals, which eventually leads to an out-of-control binge. Because they try to keep their behavior private, they have to find a time and place to binge and purge. As a result, they may become more secretive.

For those with bulimia, the need to binge and purge becomes uncontrollable and overwhelming. Clinicians diagnose a patient as having bulimia if he or she binges and purges at least twice a week for three months.

After a binge, people with bulimia feel compelled to purge to compensate for what they've eaten. Vomiting isn't the only way people who are bulimic purge. They also fast, exercise excessively, and use laxatives, diuretics, and **Ipecac syrup** in an effort not to gain weight after a binge.

Binge-eating disorder

Binge eating can happen at any time of the day or night, but many binge eaters suffer from insomnia. They do much of their binge eating late at night. Some people with the eating disorder eat in their sleep. They sleepwalk into the kitchen sometimes to binge and sometimes to eat just a small amount of food. They may eat foods in strange combinations or even raw. Some sleepwalkers prepare an entire meal. This night bingeing may happen once during the night or repeatedly. In the morning, it will probably be obvious that food was prepared and eaten. Yet the person who binged is unlikely to remember anything about the episode.

SOCIAL PATTERNS

People with eating disorders tend to become isolated. They generally have a negative self-image and their eating behaviors interfere with normal social activities. For some, food becomes their preferred source of comfort, the friend that is always there. For others, the lengths they go to avoid eating and gaining weight can be a source of strength. They often feel different and alone, unable to share their secret life with others.

TEENS SPEAK

My "Perfect Brother" Had an Eating Disorder

I have always been jealous of my older brother, Jim. He's the smart one. The popular one. The athletic one. It seems as if he's good at whatever he wants to do. So when he decided to try out for the diving team, no one doubted he would make it. Of course he did.

His coach was strict but enthusiastic about what he called my brother's "natural ability." There was just one problem. He thought Jim would be a better diver if he lost about 10 pounds. My brother, always up for a challenge, began a strict diet.

Dieting was tough for Jim, because he loved food. At first, he was very careful about what he ate, and I could see he'd lost some weight. I can't imagine anyone exercising more and eating less. I'm sure he was starved.

One day I came home late and ran into Jim just after one of his long practices. He was eating a huge sandwich, chips, and cookies. I told him if that was diet food, I wanted to be on his diet. He laughed and told me it was okay to eat such a big "snack" because he had just worked out. I didn't doubt that he was hungry but was a little surprised he was still losing weight if he was eating like that on a regular basis.

My parents could talk of nothing but diving. They went to every meet, videotaped his dives, and analyzed each one for days going over what Jim did well and what he needed to work on.

At first I thought it was cool, but little by little I started to see changes in Jim. For one thing, he got angry over really stupid things. He never seemed to be in a good mood any more. Even though he was still involved in just about everything in high school, he didn't seem to have time for fun anymore. Instead of hanging out with friends, he was always working out at the gym. He missed a lot of family meals and when he did have dinner with us, he would leave the table when he was done. He said he was going to do his homework, but instead he went to the bathroom.

I had never heard of bulimia until a friend of mine told me his sister had it. He had some pamphlets about bulimia at his house, and the more I read, the more symptoms I recognized. Could my perfect brother have bulimia? For the first time in my life, I wasn't jealous of Jim.

TESTING FOR EATING DISORDERS

To diagnose an eating disorder, health-care professionals administer a number of tests. Often the first is a thorough physical examination. It usually includes questions about eating and exercise habits and the use of laxatives or other drugs. The physician may also ask how the patient perceives his or her body. Females who have reached puberty are questioned about the regularity of their menstrual cycle.

The physical part of the examination includes a check of height and weight. The doctor will looks for physical symptoms of an eating disorder by inspecting gums and teeth, check for signs of bloating, heart rate, bone density, and levels of iron in the blood.

The doctor may suggest tests to help in a diagnosis. These tests may include checks of the **endocrine system** (glands that produce and release **hormones**), **metabolism** (the way the body creates and uses energy), and the central nervous system (the brain, spinal cord, and spinal nerves).

A urine test (urinalysis) and a blood test are part of most exams. The doctor may order a complete blood count (CBC) to see how much iron is in the blood and the number of red and white blood cells and platelets. The information gathered from these tests may point to a variety of health problems or suggest the need for furthering testing.

The doctor may also call for other blood tests to see how the liver, kidney, thyroid, pituitary gland, and ovaries are functioning.

In addition, the doctor may run an **electrocardiogram** (also called an EKG or ECG) a test to monitor heart function. In that test, electrodes are attached to the chest. The electrodes detect electrical impulses from the heart and a machine records them on a graph. (This doesn't hurt at all.) A chest X-ray may also be ordered. Anorexia may reduce the size of the heart and damage the heart muscles.

To check for damage to the brain or digestive tract, a doctor may order a computerized tomography (CT) scan. He or she may also call for a bone density test, where a sonometer sends sound waves through the bones to see how dense they are. (These tests don't hurt either.)

Fact Or Fiction?

People who have physical symptoms of an eating disorder don't need further testing.

The Facts: It's important to assess both the psychological and physical symptoms of an eating disorder in order to know the extent of the problem and to be able to treat the patient effectively.

WHAT DOCTORS CAN LEARN

Eating disorders are the focus of considerable research, because much is still unknown. Physicians are interested in learning more about the effectiveness of various combinations of treatments, including medication and therapy. Family and twin studies may reveal that some individuals are genetically predisposed to anorexia and bulimia. A number of experts are looking at the ways a highly complex nervous system with molecules that act as messengers controls appetite and energy use. By better understanding this process, they may be able to develop more effective medications.

PSYCHOLOGICAL ASSESSMENT

Eating disorders are a form of mental illness, so a thorough evaluation of symptoms includes a psychological assessment. These tests look for signs of depression and **anxiety**, poor self-image, and problems with family and other interpersonal relationships.

A psychological assessment usually begins with a clinical interview. This may be an open-ended conversation between the psychologist and the patient or it may follow a specific pattern of questioning. The assessment is likely to include one or more tests to determine the patient's state of mind and develop baseline data that can be reexamined after treatment.

The standard psychological test developed to assess an eating disorder and its severity covers a number of specific areas, assessing things like how strongly one feels the need to be thin, how satisfied one is with his or her body, **perfectionist** tendencies, fear of becoming older and more independent, and how secure one is in social situations.

EMOTIONAL RESPONSES

Many people are concerned with their weight, have a poor self-image, or have difficulty acclimating to new stages in life. So why do some people get eating disorders and others don't? There isn't an easy answer. An eating disorder is often the result of a blend of genetics, biochemical makeup (how the brain is wired), personality traits, family issues, society's expectations, personal values, and peer pressure.

FAMILY TRAITS

People with eating disorders often live with families that are overprotective, rigid, or ineffective in handling conflict, according to Anorexia Nervosa and Related Disorders, Inc. (ANRED). Those families have high expectations for achievement but provide little emotional support.

In *Eating Disorders: Everything You Need to Know*, physicians Jim Kirkpatrick and Paul Caldwell claim that obesity and alcohol abuse are common in families of people with bulimia. The families of people with anorexia also tend to be less stable than others. Childhood sex abuse has been linked to eating disorders.

PERCEPTION OF SELF

A consistent personality trait among people with eating disorders is a lack of **self-esteem** (positive feelings about oneself). People who develop a sense of self-worth in childhood are able to deal with anxious and stressful times throughout their lives. Those who don't develop a sense of self-worth during childhood often feel unhappy and worthless despite great achievement. An outsider may see a bright, straight-A student who is a leader among her peers, but she may see herself as a failure.

People with eating disorders tend to define themselves by their appearance. Their perception of themselves is inextricably linked with what they think their body looks like and how they think it should look. What they see in the mirror is often a very distorted view of reality. They never look thin enough, making it that much harder to overcome a negative self-image.

Q & A

Question: How can I help my friend who has been diagnosed with an eating disorder?

Answer: Continue being a friend. She needs you. Even though experts may be helping her recover, you can support her in many ways. Try to focus on her as a person and not how she looks or what issues she has with food. Instead of going shopping for clothes, shop for music. Instead of having lunch together, go to a movie. If she wants to talk, listen, and if she doesn't, that's okay too. Don't judge your friend and don't feign empathy if you really can't imagine how she feels. Don't be hurt if she needs time away from you. If she feels like she's not getting the support or information that she needs, suggest she go to www. nationaleatingdisorders.org or www.anred.com.

USING SYMPTOMS TO IDENTIFY A PROBLEM

Despite the fact that the symptoms of eating disorders are well-known, they are difficult to diagnose. People with eating disorders come to depend so much on their disorder that they don't want to let it go. They often go to great lengths to hide their symptoms. Also, parents and friends may not want to believe that someone they love has a problem.

See also: Anorexia; Bulimia; Depression and Weight; Laxative Abuse; Morbidity and Mortality; Purging

FURTHER READING
Kirkpatrick, Jim, M.D., and Paul Caldwell, M.D. "Eating Disorders: Everything You Need to Know." Buffalo, N.Y.: Firefly Books, 2001.

Sacker, Ira M., and Sheila Buff. *Regaining Your Self.* New York: Hyperion, 2007.

■ EATING DISORDERS IN MEN AND BOYS

Psychological disorders characterized by a compulsive obsession with food or weight. At one time, eating disorders were rarely discussed. Over the last 20 years, however, medical experts, family members, and those who have suffered from eating disorders have begun to speak openly about the problem. The result has been new research and new treatments. Yet much of the emphasis has been on women with eating disorders. Men who have the same problems have been virtually ignored.

One reason for the disproportionate attention to women with eating disorders may lie in the fact that studies have historically shown that women far outpace men when it comes to suffering from eating disorders. Those numbers may be changing, however. More boys seem to be developing eating disorders and, slowly, more boys and men are admitting to the problem and seeking treatment. Today, the issue of male eating disorders is no longer likely to be ignored.

RATES

Using the data collected by the CDC's Youth Risk Behavior Surveillance System, a research team led by Y. May Chao of Wesleyan University studied trends in teens and weight control between 1995 and 2005. In an article about the study, published in 2007 in the *International Journal of Eating Disorders*, the researchers suggest that social pressure for men to "achieve unrealistic body ideals" has increased.

Ira Sacker, director of eating disorders at Brookdale University Hospital Medical Center in Brooklyn, New York, says he has seen boys as young as nine years old with eating disorders. In the late 1990s, he estimated the ratio of female to male patients at his center dropped dramatically—from 19 to 1 to 9 to 1.

Analysis of data from the National Comorbidity Survey Replication, published in 2007 in *Biological Psychiatry*, showed that 0.3 percent of men had had anorexia, 0.5 percent of the men had had bulimia, and

2 percent of men had had binge-eating disorder at some point in their lives.

A study published in the *American Journal of Psychiatry* in 2001, "Comparisons of Men with Full or Partial Eating Disorders, Men without Eating Disorders, and Women with Eating Disorders in the Community," reports that 20 years ago researchers were likely to find one male for every 10 or 15 females with anorexia or bulimia. Now, they encounter one male with anorexia for every four females with the disorder.

The lead author of the study, D. Blake Woodside, observed that his research showed the prevalence of eating disorders among men was much closer to the prevalence among women than most people had realized, which leads to questions about why men don't seek treatment at the same rate women do.

In terms of treatment for eating disorders, males and females are anything but equal. A 1995 study done at McLean Hospital in Belmont, Massachusetts, found that only 16 percent of men with an eating disorder sought treatment. In contrast, 52 percent of the female sample went for treatment. Experts believe that men don't seek treatment as often as women because the problem isn't as socially acceptable for men, and because very few treatment programs or centers exist that are specifically designed for boys and men. One exception is Rogers Memorial Hospital in Wisconsin. In addition to its programs for girls and women, the hospital offers male-only therapy sessions and an inpatient, residential program that is exclusively male.

Fact Or Fiction?

Boys with eating disorders are usually gay.

The Facts: It's true that boys with eating disorders worry that they might be labeled as homosexual if their eating disorder is discovered. But it isn't true that only homosexuals have eating disorders. In the 1995 study done at McLean Hospital, homosexuality was not a factor in the incidence of eating disorders among the college-aged males. Some experts believe, however, that homosexuals may be more comfortable admitting to an eating disorder and seeking treatment. They warn that this could lead to data that shows a greater connection between homosexuality and eating disorders than may actually exist.

CAUSES

Many of the general causes attributed to eating disorders also explain why boys and men develop them. Depression, **anxiety**, **bipolar disorder**, and low **self-esteem** contribute to eating disorders for both males and females. A family history of eating disorders may also put boys and men at greater risk, particularly because they may see unhealthy attitudes toward food among their mothers or sisters.

In boys and men, athletics is a major contributor to the risk of developing an eating disorder. Wrestlers have a reputation for taking drastic measures to reach to a certain weight class. The desire to achieve the desired weight and peer pressure among teammates can have powerful effects. Some wrestlers may fast, exercise excessively, and wear rubber suits in an effort to drop water weight. To make matters worse, those same athletes may then eat excessively later in the year to increase their weight for a sport like football.

Wrestlers and football players aren't the only athletes worried about weight. Swimmers, track stars, jockeys, bodybuilders, rowers, gymnasts, and dancers are also at risk of developing eating disorders, according to a 1995 study, "Weight Loss, Psychological and Nutritional Patterns in Competitive Male Body Builders," by R. E. Andersen and others. In each of these sports, size can be a competitive advantage.

Media influence, which plays a role in causing anorexia and bulimia among females, is believed to be one influencing factor in a body dysmorphic disorder called bigorexia, which is also known as **muscle dysmorphia**. Researchers haven't studied this disorder very long, but it does seem that this is the only body image disorder that affects more males than females.

In magazines, movies, and on television, you're bombarded with images of waif-like women alongside men who are showing off strong arms, perfect abs, and rock-hard pecs. So it is no wonder that instead of wanting to be thinner, people suffering from bigorexia are obsessed with a desire to have bigger muscles. Like anorexics, bigorexics often don't have a realistic perception of what their body actually looks like. Even if they are muscular, they don't see themselves that way.

TEENS SPEAK

Making Weight

Ever since junior high school, I had wanted to be on the high-school wrestling team. Our wrestling team had won the state championship five years running. My older brother was on the team, and everybody in school knew his name.

When I made the wrestling team, I was instantly popular, just as I knew I would be. I loved the attention, but I loved being part of a team even more.

Workouts were tough and being a member of a winning team was both exciting and stressful. We had a lot to live up to. I probably had more to live up to than anybody. I desperately wanted to follow in my brother's footsteps and lead the team.

One day my coach told me he thought it would be better for me to wrestle in a lower weight class. His compliments were enough to pump me up. I told him losing the weight would be no problem at all. Then I went home and called my brother at college. I needed advice.

As it turned out, he knew a lot about losing weight. He gave me a regimen to follow, which included eating fruit for breakfast, salad for lunch and 16 peas for dinner for the next three nights. He told me if I chewed each pea 20 times, I would trick my body into feeling full. He was wrong. I was still hungry, but I didn't care.

I wasn't the only one worried about "making weight" at the next wrestling meet. Plenty of guys were in the same boat. I shared my brother's eating tips and they told me how to burn extra calories. We worked out like crazy, running and doing whatever we could to burn off calories. On the day of the meet, we wore three sweatshirts when we ran, and afterwards we all got under a pile of gym mats, sweating off as many calories as we could. On the bus ride over to the meet, we spit into cups (believe it or not), hoping to lose even more.

Every one of us "made weight" and qualified for our wrestling matches. After we weighed in, we had a couple hours for lunch and then we had to weigh in again. As long as we didn't go up by more than three pounds, we qualified. Naturally, we went right for the cafeteria and each of us ate a huge lunch to power up for the match.

Intellectually, I knew what we were doing wasn't healthy. Still, we were in it together and that was enough to make feeling bad feel good.

REVIEWING THE RESEARCH

The scope of research on males with eating disorders is much narrower than the research on females, but it is likely to broaden as more experts take the issue seriously. Still, a 2001 study, "Comparisons of Men with Full or Partial Eating Disorders, Men without Eating Disorders, and Women with Eating Disorders in the Community," found that men and women with eating disorders are clinically similar. Both can benefit from all of the research that has been done to date, regardless of which gender was studied.

Because no universal cause of or treatment for eating disorders exists, every person with an eating disorder—male and female—needs to be evaluated and treated individually, based on the unique characteristics of his or her case.

See also: Anorexia; Bigorexia/Muscle Dysmorphia; Binge-eating Disorder; Bulimia; Depression and Weight; Eating Disorders, Causes of; Eating Disorders, Symptoms and Diagnosis of; Media and Eating Disorders; Morbidity and Mortality; Treatment; Women and Eating Disorders

FURTHER READING

Hurley, Jennifer A., ed. *Eating Disorders: Opposing Viewpoints.* San Diego, Calif.: Greenhaven Press, 2001.

Langley, Jenny. *Boys Get Anorexia Too: Coping with Male Eating Disorders in the Family.* London: Paul Chapman Publishing, 2006.

■ ETHNICITY, GENETICS, AND EATING DISORDERS

Where you and your family are from, the race and culture with which you identify, and the characteristics you inherit from your parents. Does a black woman have a harder time controlling the urge to eat than an Asian man? Will you be more prone to anorexia because your mother suffered from it? Does a Hispanic child have greater odds of becoming bulimic than someone who isn't Hispanic? Is there such thing as a "fat gene" that predestines you to being **overweight** your entire life?

Maybe these questions sound silly to you, but scientists are very interested in figuring out why people have eating disorders—and they don't have all the answers yet. They want to know what the risk factors are that make a person more likely to get an eating disorder so that they can figure out how to prevent eating disorders from happening in the first place. Researchers are therefore looking at whether different ethnic groups share a proclivity for or tendency toward certain eating disorders. They also are comparing twins to get an idea whether eating disorders are genetic. Studies have shown that other psychiatric illnesses, including schizophrenia, depression, **anxiety**, and **obsessive-compulsive disorder**, can be inherited. Why not eating disorders? The link between ethnicity, genetics, and eating disorders is a relatively new, and important, area of research.

ETHNICITY

According to the National Eating Disorder Association (NEDA), early research and surveys on eating disorders did not include members of different ethnicities and races because of a biased belief that only white women had eating disorders. Now, researchers know that eating disorders affect women and men, girls and boys, Asian Americans, African Americans, Native Americans, Hispanics, and others. No one is immune.

NEDA says that reports of eating disorders among women of color are rising, but it's difficult to know whether the incidence of eating disorders in this group is truly increasing. It may be that they're being better represented in the research now, or that they are more apt to admit to an eating disorder now than in the past.

On its Web site, NEDA outlines a list of studies that were done in the previous decade that show ethnicity is a factor to be considered in eating disorder research. A study led by Wesleyan University researcher Ruth H. Striegel-Moore and published in 2000, for example, found that black girls are especially at risk for binge-eating.

Stereotypes may suggest that black women don't subscribe to the same thin ideal that plagues so many white women—that curves are appreciated by both women and the men they are looking to attract.

But some research shows otherwise. *Essence* magazine surveyed black women in 1994 and found that more than 70 percent of its respondents said they were "preoccupied with the desire to be thinner" and that 52 percent said they were "preoccupied with food."

Q & A

Question: As an African American woman, I feel it's important to me to be a role model to my younger siblings and other young black girls. Does that affect my risk of having an eating disorder?

Answer: A 1993 study found that African American women do feel a pressure to be role models, which also makes them feel they must be perfect. That desire for perfection is a factor that can lead to eating disorders. The same situation was described in a 1995 study of Asian and Asian American women. The researcher felt that they, too, may be more at risk for an eating disorder, particularly anorexia, because of that drive for perfection.

The compulsion to lose weight is one factor that can lead to an eating disorder. One large study, published in 1999, compared more than 6,000 adolescents and included Asians, blacks, Hispanics, Caucasians, and Native Americans. Researchers found that approximately the same percentage of Asians, blacks, Hispanics, and Caucasians had tried to lose weight, ranging between 31.9 percent and 36.1 percent. The group that stood out in the study were Native Americans. A little more than 48 percent of them had tried to lose weight—nearly half the group.

A 1997 study published in *Pediatrics* focused specifically on Native American teenagers and found similar results. More than 48 percent of girls and 30 percent of boys had dieted in the past year. The study also found that 28 percent of girls and 21 percent of boys reported purging.

A frequently cited study on Asian Americans was published in 1995 in the journal *Eating Disorders*. The researcher found that Asian and Asian American women were becoming more susceptible to eating disorders and may also be less likely to get treated for an eating disorder because they feel ashamed of what they perceive as their own weakness. Moreover, their negative attitudes toward signs of weakness may in turn exacerbate the problem, since people with eating disorders are often looking for a way to have control over their lives. Their desire to live up to a cultural ideal can also lead to perfectionism, which can lead to anorexia.

Other studies, including one published in 1996 in the *Journal of Adolescent Health*, show that Asian girls are even more likely to be unhappy with their bodies than white girls, and the less attractive they think they are, the lower their self-esteem.

In the *Journal of Adolescent Health* study, researchers reported that Hispanics are another group just as likely to be dissatisfied with their bodies. Researchers found that among the leanest 25 percent of sixth and seventh grade girls, those two groups—Asians and Hispanics—were the ones most unhappy about how their bodies looked.

One of the most recent studies on ethnicity and eating disorders was conducted by researchers at Yale University's psychiatry department and published in the journal *Eating Disorders* in 2007. The study compared black and Hispanic women to see if their body images and eating disordered behaviors were very different. In this study, while concerns about eating and depression did predict body image among the women, their ethnicity did not. There was no clear pattern that differentiated black women from Hispanic women in the study.

Similar findings were presented in *Psychology of Women Quarterly* in 2000, in a study conducted at California State University that included Hispanic, Asian, black, and white women with and without eating disorders. The researchers found that Hispanics were the most likely to use diuretics and black women most likely to use laxatives, but otherwise saw no difference among the groups when it came to presenting symptoms of bulimia, anorexia, and binge-eating disorder.

Acculturation

Some people embrace their ethnicity. The way they dress, their hairstyle, their language, and the people they look up to may be influenced by how strongly they identify with their heritage. **Acculturation** is what happens when cultures start blending. People may associate less with their ethnic or cultural identity and more with the predominant culture of the country they live in.

Eating disorders are not solely an American phenomenon, or even unique to Western cultures, but our society does seem to perpetuate the problem. As people in minority groups become more "Americanized," pulling away from their ethnic identities, they may be more at risk of eating disorders.

The reasons acculturation could be a risk factor are varied. The most obvious is that people become more aware of the thin body type associated with the American beauty standard and develop a stronger desire to embody that American standard. In addition, the stress of trying to belong to two cultures, or to move from one to the other, could be another factor, according to researchers in Australia. A 1999 study in the *Hispanic Journal of Behavioral Sciences* found that Cuban American women who strongly identified with Cuban culture were less likely to develop an eating disorder. That cultural identification may have acted as protection for them, making them less vulnerable.

A 2000 study published in the *International Journal of Eating Disorders* focused on Mexican Americans. Researchers found that second generation Mexican-American women (born in America to parents who weren't born here) were the most acculturated. They were also the most likely to exhibit disordered eating.

The tie between acculturation and eating disorders is present in other studies, as well. The California State University study described earlier, which included white, black, Hispanic, and Asian women, found that the more acculturated the women, the more likely they were to have eating disorders. On a more positive note, of those with eating disorders, the more acculturated women were more likely to receive treatment than those who were not acculturated.

It is hard to draw definitive conclusions about ethnicity and eating disorders when you review the various studies that have been done to date. Does belonging to a minority group have a tendency to make someone *more likely* to develop an eating disorder, either because of stress and societal pressure or general dissatisfaction with one's body? Or are minorities just *as likely* as Caucasians to develop an eating disorder? The evidence is inconclusive. However, the research makes one thing very clear—new studies can be expected to include more diverse populations now that scientists have shown all groups are at risk.

GENETICS

Figuring out whether eating disorders are genetic is complicated. If a study shows that daughters of women with eating disorders often get eating disorders themselves, is it because the mother passed down a gene that influences her daughter's behavior? Or is it because of the society and environment the mother and daughter both live in, which may lead to perfectionist tendencies, self-esteem issues, and other risk factors for eating disorders?

Researchers have found that genetics play a role in attitudes that lead to eating disorders (such as body dissatisfaction and preoccupation with weight), behaviors associated with eating disorders (such as bingeing, purging, and restricting calories), and eating disorders themselves. An international group of researchers has been collaborating since the mid-1990s in an attempt to unravel the ties between genetics and eating disorders, and the National Institute of Mental Health (NIMH) now funds 10 international research sites involved with this collaboration.

Some medical diseases are caused by a single gene, and once scientists determine which gene it is, they have a better chance of figuring out how to diagnose and treat that disease. In the case of eating disorders, researchers believe more than one gene is probably involved, and that genetics is only one component that increases your risk of having an eating disorder. The environment that surrounds you, the norms and values of the society you grow up in, and your genetic makeup are all involved.

A psychiatrist named Albert Stunkard, who has studied eating disorders for more than 50 years, began seriously considering the question of genetics in the 1980s. He figured out that he could look at adoption studies and twin studies to find some answers.

Adoption studies help researchers to separate environmental influences from genetic ones. Stunkard began by looking at the Danish Adoption Registry and published a paper in the *New England Journal of Medicine* in 1986 with his findings that the **body mass index (BMI)** of adopted children tended to be similar to that of their biological parents, rather than matching the BMIs of the parents who raised them. In these cases of "nature vs. nurture," nature prevailed.

In 1990 he published new findings in the same journal. This time, he had looked at the Swedish twin registry. Fraternal twins share only some of the same genes, but identical twins share all of the same genes. Comparing data between these two groups helps researchers draw conclusions about the role genes play in these disorders. Stunkard found that adult identical twins who were raised apart from one another had the same BMIs, as did identical twins who'd been raised together. The BMIs of fraternal twins were more varied, leading Stunkard to believe that genetics do influence your weight—which would also influence your predisposition to eating disorders.

Genetics and anorexia and bulimia

Walter Kaye is one of the foremost researchers in the field of genetics and eating disorders and leads the international collaborative group mentioned earlier in this chapter. When Kaye began his studies, his belief that genetics were playing a role in eating disorders stemmed from this fact: even though many people in our society are concerned about weight and influenced by the desire to have a perfect body, the percentage of our population suffering from anorexia and bulimia is still relatively small. He could not see how environmental and societal factors were solely to blame.

One of the most recent studies that includes genetics and anorexia was led by Cynthia Bulik of the University of North Carolina and published in the 2006 *Archives of General Psychiatry*. Bulik found that anorexia was passed on genetically 56 percent of the time. This is similar to the findings of other twin studies, published in 2000 and 2001, which reported that more than 50 percent of anorexia cases studied had a genetic link. Twin studies published in the 1990s reported that between 54 and 83 percent of bulimia cases also had genetics in common.

In 2003, Bulik, Kaye, and other researchers reported that they had found a specific chromosome that could be linked to self-induced vomiting common among bulimics. The study was published by the *American Journal of Human Genetics*.

Genetics and obesity

Psychiatrist Albert Stunkard, who used adoption and twin studies to find that genetics influence BMI, is now involved in an ongoing study at the University of Pennsylvania that began in 1993 with a group of 80 pregnant women, 40 of whom were obese. By age nine, half of the children of obese mothers had become obese and none of the children of lean mothers had become obese. He is continuing to follow the group and hypothesizes that he will see obesity passed on to even more of the women's children before the study is finished.

Jules Hirsch and Rudolph Leibel have also studied obesity with the intention of learning more about whether obesity is biological. In 1995 the *New England Journal of Medicine* published the results of a study they did on 41 men and women at the Rockefeller Hospital,

18 of whom were obese. It was a closely controlled hospital study in which researchers carefully controlled the subjects' diets and exercise and monitored their metabolism throughout the study. They concluded that regardless of sex, age, or ethnicity, when the obese people lost weight, their metabolism slowed down and stayed slower even after they had maintained a new weight for up to 16 weeks.

These researchers believe that you have a weight range where your particular body is comfortable, and that when you try to go too far outside that range, your body fights back by changing your appetite and your metabolism.

Jeffrey Friedman of Rockefeller University says the biological forces behind body weight can be compared to breathing. You can hold your breath for only so long before your body forces you to take a breath. He says that obese people feel an intense hunger that may not be quite as powerful as the need to breathe but is probably at least as powerful as the urge to drink when you are thirsty—requiring great willpower to resist.

Fact Or Fiction?

I inherited obesity from my parents and will just have to live with it.

The Facts: Albert Stunkard and other researchers say that despite the evidence they have gathered, showing that weight can be inherited, you should not be resigned to being overweight. Rather, it's important that you realize that reaching and maintaining a healthy weight requires vigilance throughout your lifetime, to battle the genetic predisposition. Fad diets won't work. The weight will come back. Instead, you need to develop a lifestyle that includes good nutritional choices and regular exercise.

CAN SOMEONE OF AVERAGE WEIGHT BE STARVING?

Jules Hirsch, of the Rockefeller University, studied obese women who at one time had weighed more than 200 pounds but managed, through extreme effort, to get down to normal weights. Hirsch found that even though their weight was normal, the women had symptoms of anorexia. They were obsessed with food, they were cold and tired all the time, and some stopped getting their periods. In other words, their bodies, which looked normal on the outside, were functioning internally as if they were starving.

See also: Anorexia; Bulimia; Eating Disorders, Causes of; Obesity

FURTHER READING
Fairburn, Christopher G., and Kelly D. Brownell. *Eating Disorders and Obesity, Second Edition: A Comprehensive Handbook.* New York: The Guilford Press, 2002.
Kolata, Gina. *Rethinking Thin: The New Science of Weight Loss—and the Myths and Realities of Dieting.* New York: Farrar, Straus and Giroux, 2007.

■ EXERCISE
Physical activity to develop or maintain fitness. You may think you don't have the time or energy or desire to exercise, but the benefits may encourage you to think differently. There is mounting evidence that exercise is important to overall health and well-being.

HEALTHY EXERCISE PRACTICES
Americans generally agree that exercise is good for their body. Yet exactly how much exercise is needed has been the subject of many studies and much debate.

Experts recommend the "Dietary Guidelines for Americans," published by the U.S. Department of Agriculture (USDA) and the U.S. Department of Health and Human Services (DHHS). In 2005, they suggested that children and adolescents exercise moderately for 60 minutes and adults for 30 minutes most days (and preferably every day) of the week. Walking two miles in 30 minutes is considered moderate exercise. The same is true of other activities that require about the same level of energy. Exercising at a higher intensity can reduce exercise time.

A matter of considerable debate is whether continuous activity for a particular amount of time is necessary to reap the benefits of exercise. The Dietary Guidelines say that one long exercise session or three to six shorter sessions during the day are equally beneficial.

You can add exercise to your day by choosing to do something purely for the sake of exercise, like working out at a gym, taking an exercise class, following a workout tape, running, or walking. You may prefer to play a team or individual sport. Or you may decide to participate in activities that make you sweat—dancing, hiking, biking, skating, even gardening.

You can also increase your exercise level in small ways throughout the day by choosing to walk instead of drive, parking farther from your destination, or taking the stairs instead of an elevator. Each of the active things you do in the course of a day counts toward your exercise goal.

Increasing physical fitness offers many health benefits. The USDA and DHHS cite the following rewards:

- Helps build and maintain healthy bones, muscles, and joints
- Builds endurance and muscular strength
- Helps manage weight
- Lowers **risk factors** for cardiovascular disease, colon cancer, and type 2 **diabetes**
- Helps control blood pressure
- Promotes psychological well-being and **self-esteem**
- Reduces feelings of depression and **anxiety**

In 2001 the Youth Risk Behavior Survey defined "sufficient vigorous physical activity" as participating in activities that made the students sweat and breathe hard for more than 20 minutes on at least three days during the week prior to the survey. At the time, 57 percent of females and 72.6 percent of males met the criteria.

But in 2005, the definitions changed. This time the survey asked if students had done physical activity that made them "breathe hard some of the time for a total of at least 60 minutes/day" on five or more days the week before the survey. The percentage of students meeting this new recommended level of physical activity fell considerably short. Only 27.8 percent of females and 43.8 percent of males met that goal. However, the students' overall level of exercise had gone up a little. More than 61 percent of females and nearly 76 percent of males met the 2001 standard for sufficient vigorous physical activity.

High School Student Participation in Physical Activity

	Met currently recommended levels of physical activity	Met previously recommended levels of physical activity	No vigorous or moderate physical activity
Female	27.8%	61.5%	11.3%
Male	43.8%	75.8%	7.9%

Source: Youth Risk Behavior Survey, 2005.

Burning calories

Many Internet sites have calculators that can help you figure out how many **calories** you burn during exercise. You can find one by entering "calorie counter" in the search bar at http://www.WebMD.com. iGoogle has a calorie calculator that lets you keep a running tally of calories you consume each day. How much one burns depends on the intensity of the physical activity and weight. The following table shows the number of calories a 100-pound person and a 150-pound person will burn doing various activities for 20 minutes.

	100-pound person	150-pound person
Cooking	41	61
Yoga	55	83
Walking (20-minute mile)	69	104
Gardening	70	105
Dancing (aerobic, easy)	83	124
Biking (9.4 mph)	91	136
Running ($11\frac{1}{2}$-minute mile)	123	184
Soccer	125	188
Swimming (fast crawl)	142	213
Swimming (breast stroke)	147	221

Fact Or Fiction

I'm always on the go, and I'm sure that won't change as I get older, so I don't think I really need to worry about making exercise a habit.

The Facts: Don't take your activity level for granted. Make exercise a priority in life now and you're likely to continue the habit later. If you don't, you could become an unhealthy statistic. More than half of all adults in the United States do not get enough physical activity and one quarter of adults don't use their leisure time for physical activity, according to a national phone survey conducted in 2005 by the Centers for Disease Control and Prevention.

TEENS SPEAK

My Exercise Wake-Up Call

I used to hate exercising. I tried jogging, aerobics, team sports. You name it. I usually started each exercising adventure with a friend, but I never lasted very long and didn't really worry about it much. And I wasn't the only one. Since middle school, most of my friends and I were spending more energy devising ways to avoid physical education class than we have participating. It wasn't as if we were sitting around all the time—we were involved in a bunch of clubs and activities. I wasn't fat and ate pretty much whatever I wanted, so I figured I was in okay shape.

Then one day, I came home to find an ambulance outside our door. My father had had a heart attack while goofing around in the pool with my little brother. He was only 47. After that, the doctor taught my dad about the importance of physical fitness, and the whole family got the message. I finally admitted that exercise was important, but I was pretty busy with school and friends and had to really think about how I would fit it in.

Everything came together after a talk with my guidance counselor. We were talking about college, which seemed very far off since I was just a freshman. She mentioned that she had just started a rowing club, because a number of colleges have great rowing scholarships. The early morning practices sounded a little harsh, but I promised her I'd give it a try.

Two years later, I'm still rowing. I actually love being out on the water early in the morning. It starts out peaceful and cool. Then we start to row. We all get this rhythm going and it's pretty amazing. Even though I get up earlier, rowing practice energizes me for the whole day.

As it turns out, I'm pretty good. I don't know if I'll get a college scholarship, but I think I have a chance. I'm definitely healthier. And I have a whole new group of friends.

ABNORMAL EXERCISE PRACTICES

The message is everywhere: exercise is good for your body, self-esteem, and social life. But too much of a good thing can be bad. **Compulsive exercise** doesn't get the attention that eating disorders do, but it is a serious disorder. Some people call it obligatory exercise or anorexia athletica. Compulsive exercisers are usually obsessed with what they look like and often have an eating disorder. Sometimes, people with bulimia will follow a **binge** with compulsive exercise, using it as a form of purging.

How much exercise is too much? Doctors have difficulty with that question. The general consensus is that when someone puts exercise before other important elements of his or her life, he or she has a problem. For example, the hours spent exercising each day may keep a person from enjoying time with friends, doing schoolwork, and even sleeping. Exercise becomes a compulsion when it is something that one has to do, no matter what the consequences or what else may be going on in his or her life. People suffering from bigorexia—who constantly worry about the size of their muscles—are often compulsive exercisers.

Compulsive exercisers often lie about how much time they spend exercising. Some exercise in private or late at night. Although it may be hard to spot the problem if someone is hiding or lying about it, some of these behaviors should make you suspicious:

- Exercising even when sick or injured
- Exercising outside in extreme weather and
- Becoming angry when asked to cut back on exercise

Q & A

Question: Can I become addicted to exercise? How can I know if I'm an exercise addict?

Answer: Researchers are still trying to figure out if exercise is addictive. They say that strenuous exercise for a long period of time releases endorphins in your body that are similar to morphine. They are not yet sure whether it's possible to become physiologically addicted to that substance. If you enjoy exercising, then you probably are not an addict. If exercise is something you feel compelled to do in order to avoid guilt and anxiety, you might have a problem. If family and friends say you're overdoing it, take their concern seriously.

Like eating disorders, compulsive exercise is a mental illness that has severe physical consequences. Girls who exercise too much can throw their **hormones** out of balance and change their menstrual cycle or stop it entirely. The combination of extreme amounts of exercise and poor nutrition is especially harmful. If a body does not get enough energy from food, it will start breaking down muscle for the energy it needs.

People who exercise compulsively may experience **dehydration**, broken bones, torn ligaments, joint problems, osteoporosis, and even heart and kidney failure. A healthy amount of exercise builds muscle, but too much actually destroys the muscle.

Fact Or Fiction?

Ordinary people can exercise too much, but if you aspire to be a world-class athlete, there's no such thing as training too much.

The Facts: World-class athletes are models of discipline and hard work. Therefore it can be especially hard to tell if a competitive athlete is overdoing exercise and dieting. But some athletes do. Gymnasts, cross country runners, wrestlers, and swimmers are among the most susceptible. Although they may win championships, eventually unhealthy practices will take a serious toll on their bodies, causing grave illness or even death. So, yes, there is such a thing as training too much.

WEIGHT AND PHYSICAL ACTIVITY

Physical activity is not only important for overall health but also a critical element in maintaining a **healthy weight** or losing weight in a healthy way. Exercise can burn calories, firm and tone muscles, and strengthen the body.

Aerobics

Exercise is an important component to weight control. By burning calories through exercise, you are able to eat more and therefore add more nutrients to your diet. If you have lost weight and are trying to maintain the weight loss, you're likely to need more than the minimum recommended amount of exercise.

Rena Wing, a professor of psychiatry at Brown Medical School in Providence, R.I., helped develop the National Weight Control Registry in 1994, which tracks more than 5,000 American adults who have lost an average of more than 65 pounds and kept it off for more than five years. Ninety percent of the people on the registry exercise for about an hour a day.

Aerobic exercise speeds up the heart rate and breathing. It is good for the heart and helps burn calories. Your body uses those calories for the energy it needs to keep your heart and lungs pumping faster. How many calories you burn during cardiovascular exercise depends on how much you weigh and the intensity level you maintain during the exercise.

Body sculpting

Along with burning calories, you should do exercises that increase strength and flexibility. Exercises that strengthen the body help build and maintain bones, decreasing the risk of osteoporosis (progressive loss of bone density). Strength exercises may be done with weights or weight machines, or by using your own body as resistance. Repetitive activities that require strength, such as carrying the groceries, count, too.

The more muscle in your body, the more calories you burn. Muscle weighs more than fat. So, when you build muscle through exercise, your weight may not drop, even though your body looks more toned and fit. How you look and feel is much more important than the number you see on the scale.

Stretching, dancing, yoga, and pilates are ways to increase flexibility. Increased flexibility will make your muscles longer and leaner and decrease the likelihood of injury from exercise.

Q & A

Question: I've been exercising all year and I feel really good about my improved fitness level and how my body looks. But I've gained weight! How can that be?

Answer: With all the exercise you've been doing, you've been replacing fat with muscle. The proof is in the way you look and the fact that you're stronger than you were before. Muscle weighs more than fat. So the rising number on your scale may show that you're more muscular than you were before. Unless you've beefed up enough to be a professional body builder, your body mass index (BMI) is still in the healthy range. So don't worry about the scale; be proud of how good you feel.

EXERCISE BENEFITS

Regular exercise makes most people look better, but more important it improves their physical and mental health. They don't just look better, they feel better.

See also: Bigorexia/Muscle Dysmorphia; Caloric Intake and Expenditures; Depression and Weight; Obesity; Weight Control

FURTHER READING

Kaehler, Kathy. *Teenage Fitness: Get Fit, Look Good and Feel Great!* New York: HarperResource, 2001.

■ FAD DIETS

An eating regimen that recommends or excludes a specific food or type of food. The diet may be based on the theory that some foods or combination of foods can change your body chemistry. All fad diets promise fast and easy weight loss: "Lose 20 pounds and three dress sizes in two weeks!" "Imagine your extra pounds just melting off while you sleep!" "Shhh. The miracle weight loss food that celebrities are keeping secret!" "I used to be fat, but now look at me!" "Lose weight without dieting!" These are the kinds of claims that are used to promote fad diets.

If you have ever struggled with your weight, you know how hard it can be to resist trying the latest diet. Although you know that a diet of grapefruit and hot dogs isn't nutritionally sound, you wonder what harm it can do to try it out for a couple of weeks and see if it works.

The fact is that if it sounds too good to be true, it probably is. Healthy weight loss isn't easy. Diets that promise quick weight loss are gimmicks. You may lose some water weight; you may even lose some actual weight; but the chances of keeping the weight off are poor. More importantly, fad diets endanger health by robbing the body of important nutrients, especially for those who are still growing.

Fact Or Fiction?

Certain foods, like grapefruit and cabbage soup, can burn fat.

The Facts: There are no foods that burn fat. The way to burn fat is through exercise. Some foods that contain caffeine can speed up your metabolism for a short period of time, but they will not cause you to lose weight. The way to lose weight is to use more calories than you eat.

TYPES OF FAD DIETS

People learn about fad diets from books, magazines, TV, Web sites, and word-of-mouth. These diets have had a major effect on the food industry. Fat-free cookies and low-carbohydrate nutrition bars are just two of the many special foods that manufacturers have put on the market in response to fad diets. Some restaurants even prepare special dishes or offer special combinations of foods to meet the requirements of these diets. Just because these foods are available does not mean that the diets are safe. In fact, in 2007, the theme of the American Dietetic Association's National Nutrition Month was "Be 100% Fad Free."

The magic-food diets

Many fad diets are based on one or more "magic" foods. The ads claim that if you eat this food or group of foods, you'll lose weight. Bananas, cabbage soup, grapefruit, and other foods have taken on mythical status as the means to a quick weight loss. You may even know someone who has been on one of these diets and lost weight.

When people go on diets like the Cabbage Soup Diet, they tend to get bored. So if they stick to the diet, they eat less food and fewer calories and lose weight. They also starve their body of the nutrients it needs to keep healthy. Eventually, they get so bored that they break the diet, eating more calories than they probably did before starting it. Once they go off the diet, the weight comes back.

High-protein, low-carbohydrate diets

High-protein, low-carbohydrate diets, such as the Atkin's Diet and the South Beach Diet, are popular. They are also controversial, because they do not follow recommendations made by the U.S. Department of Agriculture, the American Heart Association, the American Dietetic Association, and the American Diabetes Association. Experts from these organizations argue that it is not nutritionally sound to eliminate most carbohydrates from your diet, because doing so will deprive your body of important nutrients. A lack of carbohydrates can result in a state of **ketosis**, a condition that can make you feel tired, constipated, or nauseous. The long-term effects of ketosis include heart disease, kidney damage, and bone loss.

The same experts caution that not all carbohydrates are equally healthy. For example, foods made from fiber-rich whole grains provide more nutrition than foods made from processed white flour. The experts also believe that some high-protein, low-carbohydrate diets contain too much fat, which is dangerous to the heart, but the research is not definitive. One study, "A Randomized Trial of a Low-Carbohydrate Diet for Obesity," published in *The New England Journal of Medicine* in May 2003, found that those who followed a low-carbohydrate diet improved their **cholesterol** levels and therefore reduced the **risk factors** associated with coronary heart disease.

Another study, conducted by the Harvard School of Public Health and published in the *New England Journal of Medicine* in 2006, looked at the diet of more than 80,000 women and found that those whose diets were low in carbohydrates and high in protein and fat did not have a higher risk of heart disease.

Q & A

Question: My uncle was overweight until he went on a low-carbohydrate diet earlier this year. Now, his doctor says he's at a healthy weight. Isn't that a good thing?

Answer: Experts disagree on the benefits of low-carbohydrate diets, but if your uncle is being monitored by a doctor and feels okay, then it may be fine for him. The bigger question is whether he'll be able to maintain his new weight. "A Randomized Trial of a Low-Carbohydrate Diet for Obesity," a May 2003 study published in *The New England Journal of Medicine*, compared subjects following a low-carbohydrate diet and subjects following a low-fat diet. Researcher found that the low-carbohydrate group lost more weight during the first six months, but after a year, there was no difference in weight loss between the two groups. Both groups had difficulty staying on the diets.

High-fiber, low-calorie diets
These diets emphasize foods rich in fiber—an ingredient in vegetables, fruits, beans, and whole grains that aids in digestion. Fiber tends to make you feel full, and that feeling of fullness may leave you feeling more satisfied after a meal than you are likely to feel on a low-calorie diet. But the American Dietetic Association (ADA) warns that eating too much fiber—more than 50 or 60 grams a day—can cause cramping, bloating, and diarrhea.

Meal-replacement diets
The ADA says that using an over-the-counter diet product that replaces a meal with a nutrient-packed shake or bar can be useful for short-term weight loss, if done under a doctor's supervision. The association warns, however, that most dieters plateau after three months on such a plan. Although they may or may not lose weight, their wallet definitely gets lighter after paying for expensive meal-replacement products.

Margo Maine, author of *Body Wars: Making Peace with Women's Bodies* (2000), says that people on meal replacement diets have a 95 percent chance of regaining the weight that they lost within one to two years. For long-term weight management, she advises dieters to develop healthy eating habits.

Fasting
Some people claim that routine fasting cleanses toxins from their body. It does not. Instead, fasting can result in a loss of muscle mass, a lowered **metabolism**, and a body that stores fat more easily. At best, dieters lose water weight and feel light-headed, dizzy, and lethargic. At worst, they begin to build up **ketones**, chemical substances that

the body produces when it doesn't have enough **insulin**. A buildup of ketones can damage the kidneys.

MEDIA PROMOTION

In September 2002, the Federal Trade Commission (FTC) issued a report analyzing weight-loss advertising. The report notes that at any given time 70 percent of all Americans are trying to lose weight or keep from gaining weight. They spend more than $30 billion annually on weight-loss products. In other words, the health and diet industry taps a huge market—and they do it mainly through the media.

To compile its report, the FTC analyzed 300 ads that ran mainly in the first half of 2001. Those ads appeared on broadcast and cable television and radio as well as in magazines, newspapers, supermarket tabloids, flyers sent by direct mail, commercial e-mail (spam), and through Internet sites. The study also compared ads that ran in eight national magazines between 1992 and 2001. Researchers concluded that much of today's diet and nutrition advertising is misleading. They also noted that the number of ads more than doubled and the number of different types of ads tripled over that time period.

The FTC's findings suggest that ads in the media be viewed with caution. Nearly 40 percent of the ads in the sample "made at least one representation that almost certainly is false" and 55 percent "made at least one representation that is very likely to be false or, at the very least, lacks adequate substantiation." The FTC concluded that consumers need to be particularly wary of common techniques used to market health and weight-loss products. Nearly all of the ads the FTC studied involved at least one (and sometimes several) of these misleading techniques:

- Consumer testimonials and before-and-after pictures
- Rapid weight-loss claims
- Promises that no diet or exercise is required
- Claims of long-term or permanent weight loss
- Claims that the product is clinically proven or doctor approved
- Claims that the product provides natural or safe weight loss

Several months after issuing the report, the FTC asked the media to be more vigilant and reject any advertisements that used one or more of these techniques. In 2005, the FTC issued a report that found the incidence of these techniques in weight-loss advertising had gone from 49 percent in 2001 to 15 percent in 2004.

Media as an information source

The ADA conducted a popular-opinion survey called *Nutrition and You: Trends 2002*. Its findings suggest that consumers get more nutrition information from the media than anywhere else. The three most popular sources are television and magazines, cited by 72 percent and 58 percent of the respondents respectively, and newspapers, cited by 33 percent. The Internet, used by 13 percent of respondents, and radio, relied on by 18 percent, was less influential than other media sources. Among non-media sources of information, doctors and family and friends were relied on by about 17 percent of the respondents and doctors by 12 percent.

In the ADA's survey, women were more likely to get their information from magazines and books, and men were more likely to get their information from the radio. They also found that the older you are, the less likely you are to use the Internet or family and friends as information sources, and the more likely you are to get information from the newspaper.

The Internet is clearly a growing source of information on health and nutrition. A 2006 Harris Interactive poll said that the number of people who went online for health information rose from 117 million in 2005 to 136 million in 2006, or from 72 percent to 80 percent of Americans. Harris Interactive calls these people "cyberchondriacs."

In the past, the ADA has found that some Americans are confused by dietary advice based on new studies. One of the reasons for their confusion is the rush to report preliminary findings. As a cautious media consumer, you should question how a study was conducted, who conducted it, how many people were involved in the study, whether other studies support its findings, and who stands to gain from the study's findings.

The International Food Information Council cites another problem with the way research on diet and nutrition are reported. The group notes that news reporters, who are limited by airtime or print space, rarely provide consumers with enough context to interpret the nutritional advice they provide. They often leave out important details, including how much more or less of a food to eat, how often to eat it, and to whom the advice applies.

Where Americans get their nutritional advice, and who they trust to give it to them, are not always the same—according to the American Dietetic Association.

Identifying bad nutritional advice

Testimonials, hype, and seemingly scientific claims can easily trick people into believing a fad diet works. The Food and Nutrition Science Alliance (FANSA) suggests that you think twice before taking nutritional advice that include these red flags:

- Recommendations that promise a quick fix
- Dire warnings of dangers from a single product or regimen
- Claims that sound too good to be true
- Simplistic conclusions drawn from a complex study
- Recommendations based on a single study
- Dramatic statements that are refuted by reputable scientific organizations
- Lists of "good" and "bad" foods
- Recommendations made to help sell the product
- Recommendations based on studies published without peer review
- Recommendations from studies that ignore differences among individuals or groups

DID YOU KNOW?

Where Americans Get Nutrition Information

Television: 72%
Magazines: 58%
Newspapers: 33%
Radio: 18%
Family and friends: 17%
Internet: 13%
Doctors: 12%

Source: Nutrition and You: Trends 2002, American Dietetic Association.

TEENS SPEAK

My Perfect Prom Dress Was One Size Too Small

It was two weeks until prom, and I was on top of the world. I had a very cool boyfriend, Jay, and our friends were sure we'd be picked prom king and queen. I acted as if I didn't care one way or another, but in reality, I couldn't stop thinking about it. I live in a small town and people remember you for things like this. This was the ultimate high school fantasy, as far as I was concerned.

At first it was fun to look through magazines and search for the perfect dress for the perfect night. I spent days shopping. Finally, I found it. A dress I loved. No other dress would do. If only the dress weren't one size too small.

What I loved about the dress—that it was different, something you wouldn't see everywhere else—was also what I hated about it, because I couldn't find the dress in my size anywhere.

There was only one thing to do: diet. The ads were everywhere for quick diets that promised you would lose at least one dress size in just weeks. So I chose a diet I thought I could stick to, bought the dress, and found a friend willing to diet with me.

The first day wasn't hard. In fact, I felt great about myself for following the diet perfectly. The second day was a little harder, but I distracted myself by keeping busy. The third day I woke up with a headache. My friend wasn't feeling great either, but we convinced each other to keep going. We were both happy to see our weight dropping. By day four, my friend complained of a stomach ache and quit the diet. She had bought a dress that fit, unlike me.

As the days passed, my mother started to worry about me and threatened to take the dress back. I wouldn't hear of it. Still I had to admit (but only to myself) that I really wasn't feeling well at all.

The day before prom, I tried on the dress and it fit. And guess what? Jay and I won. Yet it wasn't the dream I imagined, because I was sick the whole night. I was tired and my stomach hurt. More than once, I got angry with Jay over stupid things. You probably aren't surprised to know that the dress doesn't fit anymore. I never want to worry about being that thin again.

THE CASE AGAINST FAD DIETS

At any age, **yo-yo dieting**—going on and off diets—is not a good way to manage your weight. People on yo-yo diets lose weight quickly, regain the lost pounds (and often more), and then try the same or a new quick weight-loss plan. Unfortunately, each time they drastically cut calories, their body goes into starvation mode, slowing down their metabolism and storing fat more easily.

Gradual weight-loss, exercise, and a healthy lifestyle are the best way to reach a **healthy weight**. Gradual weight-loss plans include a variety of foods and are designed to help most people lose a half of a pound to two pounds a week. If you have any question about whether a particular weight-loss plan is healthy, discuss it with your doctor.

See also: Caloric Intake and Expenditures; Diet Pills; Nutrition and Nutritional Deficiencies; Weight Control

FURTHER READING

Kirby, Jane, R.D., and American Dietetic Association. *Dieting for Dummies.* New York: For Dummies, 2003.

Maine, Margo, Ph.D. *Body Wars: Making Peace with Women's Bodies.* Carlsbad, Calif.: Gurze Books, 2000.

■ FOOD ALLERGIES

A negative reaction by the body's **immune system** to a food that is harmless to most people. The response to the food has to involve the immune system to be considered an allergy.

Many people have negative reactions to foods that do not involve their immune system; these are not food allergies but rather food intolerance. Lactose intolerance is a good example. Although people who are lactose intolerant have a negative reaction to dairy products, their reaction does not affect their immune system. People with lactose intolerance do not have enough lactase, an enzyme used to digest lactose or milk sugar. Food poisoning can also be confused with an allergic reaction. In a case of food poisoning, the negative reaction is a result of toxins in the food itself, not in the way the body reacts to the food. People can also have psychological reactions to certain foods.

Do some foods make you sneeze, cramp, feel nauseous, or break out in hives? Do you have difficulty breathing after eating some foods? If so, you may be among the small percentage of Americans who suffer from food allergies. Or you may be among the much larger population of people who believe they have food allergies.

True food allergies affect only four to eight percent of young children (many of whom grow out of their allergies) and less than two percent of the general population. Yet about one-third of all adults think they have a food allergy, according to statistics cited by the International Food Information Council Foundation (IFIC) in June 2001.

If a reaction to a nontoxic food can't be traced to the immune system, metabolic system, an illness, or a psychological problem, it's called a "food idiosyncrasy." One of the most common food idiosyncrasies is sulfite sensitivity. Sulfites are preservatives used most commonly in wine and dried fruits and vegetables. People who are sensitive to sulfite can have such severe reactions that the Food and Drug Administration (FDA) requires that sulfites be identified on all packaged foods. It also bans the use of sulfites on all fresh fruits and vegetables, except potatoes. People with sulfite sensitivity have reactions that range from shortness of breath to fatal shock. Some experience severe asthma attacks when exposed to sulfites.

The best way to determine if you have a food allergy is to consult an allergist.

Q & A

Question: What are the most common causes of food allergies?

Answer: Eight foods—milk, eggs, fish, soy, shellfish, wheat, peanuts, and nuts that grow on trees (such as walnuts)—are responsible for 90 percent of all allergic reactions, according to a Food and Agriculture Organization report on food allergies presented in November 1995.

IDENTIFYING ALLERGIES

Food allergies start with an allergen—the part of the food that triggers a negative response in the immune system. Most **allergens** are **proteins** and a single food can have more than one allergen. In response to the allergen, the body's immune system fights back by producing **antibodies** that make their way to the bloodstream and body tissues. The cells that carry the antibodies were making and storing **histamines**. When they encounter allergens, they release those histamines, which then cause such allergic symptoms as rashes, runny noses, and wheezing. (Now you know why some allergy medications are called antihistamines.)

The symptoms of food allergies usually appear on the skin, in the gastrointestinal tract, or in the respiratory system. Skin irritations can include itching, hives, eczema, and redness. Symptoms related to the gastrointestinal tract usually start with itching or a swelling of the lips, mouth, and throat. When the food hits the stomach, new symptoms develop, including nausea, vomiting, cramping, and diarrhea. Respiratory symptoms such as sneezing, runny nose, shortness of breath, and difficulty breathing may also develop. For those with asthma, a food allergy can trigger asthmatic symptoms. Sometimes, different parts of the body react to the allergen at the same time. This severe and sometimes even deadly reaction is called **anaphylaxis**.

One of the difficulties in diagnosing a food allergy is that the reaction may not take place at the time the food is eaten. It can happen even days later. Sensitivity to an allergen also varies greatly. One person may not even have to ingest an allergenic food. Touching it is enough to cause a reaction. Others experience symptoms only when the food is eaten in large quantities.

To diagnose a food allergy, an allergist starts by asking questions about the food that may be causing a problem. The doctor wants to know how much food is ingested before a reaction occurs, how long it takes before there is a reaction to the food, and how often reactions occur. They ask patients to keep a food diary and record symptoms so that they can figure out why there is a problem with a particular food. Patients may also undergo a physical examination to make sure that an underlying medical condition isn't misdiagnosed as an allergy.

One of the best ways to determine whether a person has a food allergy is to stop eating foods suspected of causing a reaction. Doctors call this an "elimination diet." After observing symptoms (or hopefully a lack of symptoms) over several weeks, a patient may be asked to reintroduce the suspicious foods one at a time and record if and when symptoms reoccur. Although it sounds like a simple process, elimination diets require a physician's supervision to make sure that patients continue to eat a healthy diet and to evaluate symptoms objectively. Allergists also test reactions to certain food allergens by pricking the skin and exposing it to mild solutions containing allergenic foods. They may also administer a special blood test that can help diagnose food allergies.

The allergist looks at all of the information gathered to determine whether there is a food allergy and if so, how severe it is. If the reaction isn't severe, the allergist may have a patient eat various amounts of the food to determine how much he or she can eat without triggering a reaction. Sometimes a physician will disguise the allergenic food to make sure the reaction is a physical and not an emotional response.

Q & A

Question: Can a food allergy cause emotional symptoms instead of physical symptoms?

Answer: According to some research, a "food-induced allergy" can cause emotional reactions to certain foods. For example, a person may become extremely angry, depressed, or paranoid after eating a particular food. If the food is eliminated from the diet, these extreme emotions disappear. These theories are difficult to test, making this area of research controversial.

TREATING ALLERGIES

If you are allergic to pollen, dog hair, or mold, an allergist can give you medication to prevent the symptoms or shots that will make you less sensitive to the allergen over time. Those treatments are not possible for those who have food allergies. The only way to treat the allergy is by eliminating the food from your diet—and that may sound easier than it is.

Those who have food allergies must read labels carefully and ask questions before ordering food at a restaurant or eating dinner at a friend's house. Not all foods are prepared the same way. Many allergenic foods, such as eggs, wheat, and dairy products, may be hidden in other foods. People with allergies should also become fluent in "label language." For example, *albumin* is the white of an egg. Durum semolina and farina are wheat flour. Both casein and sodium casein-ate are dairy products even though sodium caseinate may be found in some "nondairy" foods.

Those with severe sensitivities may have to be careful about food preparation. If a safe food is prepared on a surface that previously contained an allergenic food, it may cause a reaction.

Even with extreme care, mistakes happen. It is therefore wise to take precautions. To protect against anaphylaxis, an allergist can prescribe syringes filled with epinephrine, a drug used to treat severe allergic reactions, and teach a patient how to use them if necessary. It's also a good idea for people with food allergies to wear a medical alert bracelet, so that emergency personnel will know how to help them if they are unconscious.

Fact Or Fiction?

Once a food allergy is diagnosed, you have to avoid that food for the rest of your life.

The Facts: Children who are allergic to some foods, like milk or soy, often grow out of their allergy after avoiding the allergens for several years. A 1989 study published in the *Journal of Allergy and Clinical Immunology*, "Role of the Elimination Diet in Adults with Food Allergies," and a similar study on children published the same year by the *Journal of Pediatrics* showed that one-third of participants outgrew their sensitivity after one or two years following strict elimi-nation diets. Children are much less likely to grow out of an allergy to peanuts, tree nuts, fish, or shellfish. If you've been avoiding an allergenic food since childhood and want to see if you have outgrown the allergy, you should make an appointment with a professional allergist.

TAKING FOOD ALLERGIES SERIOUSLY

Mild food allergies are inconvenient, but severe food allergies are life threatening. People with food allergies must take great care to avoid certain foods and find out what ingredients may be hidden in dishes that others have prepared. Since sensitivities to allergens may change over time, people with food allergies should maintain regular contact with an allergist.

See also: Nutrition and Nutritional Deficiencies

■ FOOD AND GENDER

See: Eating Disorders in Men and Boys; Women and Eating Disorders

■ THE INTERNET AND EATING DISORDERS

A huge worldwide network of computers, the World Wide Web was developed by Tim Berners-Lee in 1991 to allow users to view documents transmitted via the Internet without downloading them. Thanks to the Internet, you can look up information on just about anything, anytime—including eating disorders. You don't have to get to a bookstore or a library. You don't have to call or make an appointment with an expert. You can do your own research, and you can find communities of people with the same concerns or interests you have, with very little effort at all.

The Internet stands apart from other information sources in two particular ways: it's accessible 24/7 and it's interactive. You can do more than just find information. You can exchange information with others. For people who have eating disorders or are at risk of having eating disorders, the Internet can be both helpful and dangerous.

INTERNET USE AMONG TEENS

Teens may be the most sophisticated users of the Internet. The Kaiser Family Foundation reported that in 2005, 74 percent of eight- to 18-year-olds had access to the Internet at home and that about half used the Internet to learn more about their health. But they are not just looking things up on the Internet. The Pew Internet & American Life Project released a study in 2005 that showed 57 percent of teens online, amounting to about 12 million people, create content for the Internet to communicate and express themselves. They create Web pages, blogs, and videos. Some of those teens create Web sites about their eating disorders.

Q & A

Question: How popular are pro-eating disorders Web sites?

Answer: According to a *Time* article from the summer of 2005, one popular site had received more than 85,000 hits in about two years. In January 2008, the counter on the site showed more than 671,000 hits. Studies show these sites are getting plenty of traffic, often by people who visit over and over.

HOW THE INTERNET HURTS: PRO-EATING DISORDERS WEB SITES

Some of the eating disorders Web sites created by teens and others are called "pro-ana" or "pro-mia" sites, with *Ana* and *Mia* serving as shorthand for *anorexia* and *bulimia*. Using pretty names for life-threatening disorders is one of the first clues that these sites are dangerous.

There are also pro-recovery sites created by eating disorder associations and recovery centers who are trying to increase awareness of and treatment for eating disorders. Many of these groups have spoken out against the pro-eating disorders sites and tried to have them removed from the Internet. While some have been removed, most are still there, and they are very easy to find. In 2003, researchers estimated that there were around 500 pro-eating disorders sites—five times as many as pro-recovery sites.

Pro-eating disorders sites may be appealing to people with eating disorders for many reasons. People with eating disorders generally try to hide their behavior, and these sites offer them a place where they do not have to hide. They can even read blogs and communicate with other people trying to lose unhealthy amounts of weight. They find information, support, and acceptance whenever they need it. If they are competitive **perfectionists**, as many people with eating disorders are, these Web sites give them an opportunity to "get better" at being anorexic, and to brag about how much weight they have lost or how good they have gotten at hiding their behavior from those who criticize them.

Generally, the creators of pro-eating disorders sites consider bingeing, purging, and starvation to be lifestyle choices rather than symptoms of serious physical and mental disorders. Go to these sites and you can learn about new ways of purging, get advice on how to hide your eating disorder from others, and much more. Many of these sites offer what they call "thinspiration," which includes quotes, poems, and many, many pictures that glorify extreme weight loss.

These sites are not necessarily out to recruit people. In fact, some have warnings discouraging people who do not have or are trying to recover from an eating disorder from entering. Instead, the creators of these sites consider them places of refuge for people with eating disorders, people who are misunderstood or judged by their families and friends. Many sites are defensive and angry, saying that they don't teach people how to have eating disorders or trigger the onset of eating disorders.

But health professionals generally disagree. They are very concerned about these sites and their potential to push someone who may be prone to an eating disorder into actually having one. They also worry that the information found on these sites may prolong disordered eating among people already suffering from an eating disorder.

Fact Or Fiction?

Pro-ana Web sites are misunderstood and unfairly maligned by people who just don't understand what it's like to be anorexic.

The Facts: That can't be true, because recovering anorexics are among those who have criticized pro-ana sites. Even if the creators of these sites say that they discourage people from becoming anorexic, the very fact that the sites exist seems to normalize behaviors that can ultimately cost you your life.

USING THE INTERNET TO HELP: PRO-RECOVERY SITES

For those who are interested in overcoming an eating disorder, there is plenty of support and information to be found on the Internet. Pro-recovery sites, including those listed in the Hotlines and Help

Sites section of this book, can help you recognize warning signs, find treatment centers, and learn about the causes behind eating disorders. Through statistics and personal anecdotes, they show people with eating disorders that they are not alone, and they offer online support forums so that information can be exchanged. They also do advocacy work, promoting more eating disorders research and health care coverage.

In 2006 researchers at Stanford University published the first major study looking at how young people (ages 10–22) with eating disorders use both pro-eating disorders sites and pro-recovery sites. They were surprised to find significant overlap. Forty-one percent visited pro-recovery sites and 35 percent visited pro-eating disorders sites, but 25 percent visited both. It may be that some people with eating disorders crave as much information as they can find about the subject, regardless of what perspective the information is coming from. Before the Internet existed, people with eating disorders were voracious readers of books about eating disorders, according to Something Fishy, a pro-recovery site.

The Stanford study found that 96 percent of those studied reported that they learned new ways to purge or lose weight on the pro-eating disorders sites. This is just what health professionals worry about. However, the study also found that 46 percent of the respondents learned new techniques for purging and weight loss from the pro-recovery sites. One of the researchers speculated that this could be because people with eating disorders have a distorted view that allows them to focus on the things that they want to hear and ignore the negative information. For example, they may ignore the overall message in an anecdote about how sick someone got from purging and instead come away with new information on how to purge without getting caught.

The Stanford researchers expected to find the people visiting pro-eating disorders Web sites to be in worse health than those visiting pro-recovery sites and that did not turn out to be the case. However, those frequenting the pro-eating disorders sites did report spending less time on schoolwork and were ill for longer periods of time. Users of both types of sites spent more time in the hospital than those who didn't visit these sites.

- Because many people with eating disorders are ashamed of their behavior and are reluctant to talk about it openly or seek help, it makes sense that the Internet also has the potential to be helpful. People who will not directly ask for information or help can instead seek it out anonymously on the Internet.

There are many sites that are not solely about eating disorders that offer good nutritional advice and can support your effort to live a healthy lifestyle. MyPyramid.gov is one example. It allows you to put in personal information and get personalized recommendations for adopting a well-balanced diet. WebMD is another site that is full of information promoting healthy habits.

The Internet may also be used therapeutically. In a study funded by the National Institute of Mental Health and published in 2006 in *Archives of General Psychiatry*, 480 college-age women identified as being at risk for developing eating disorders in San Diego and the San Francisco Bay Area were enrolled in a randomized, controlled trial of an eight-week Internet intervention program. As part of the trial, the women were given materials to read, kept an online body-image journal, and participated in an online discussion group. Researchers then interviewed the women when the eight weeks were up and again each year for up to three years.

The Internet intervention program turned out to be most success-ful with overweight women. None of these women developed eating disorders after two years, whereas nearly 12 percent of women with similar BMIs in a control group (women who didn't take part in the online trial program) developed eating disorders in the same time period. Another successful result of the intervention program: among women who started out the study already exhibiting some symptoms of an eating disorder (such as purging or exercising excessively), only 14 percent of the intervention group developed an eating disor-der within two years, compared to 30 percent of the control group. For these two groups of women, at least, participating in the online program helped to change their attitudes about weight and body image.

SOCIAL NETWORKS

Social networks seem to be the "next big thing" when it comes to sharing feelings about eating disorders. MySpace, Facebook, and YouTube all have pro-ana and pro-mia forums, along with forums speaking out just as adamantly against them. Will eating disorder researchers begin studying social networks next?

See also: Anorexia; Bulimia; Media and Eating Disorders; Nutrition and Nutritional Deficiencies; Peer Pressure; Self-Image; Women and Eating Disorders

FURTHER READING
Goodman, Laura J., and Mona Villapiano. *Eating Disorders: The Journey to Recovery Workbook.* New York: Brunner-Routledge, 2001.
CRC Health Group. Something Fishy: Website on Eating Disorders. URL: http://www.something-fishy.org.

■ LAXATIVE ABUSE
The misuse of substances that stimulate bowel movements. Abusing or misusing laxatives can cause serious medical problems.

OVER-THE-COUNTER DRUGS
Laxatives are easily obtained. If you walk into any drugstore, you'll find an array of choices: pills, capsules, liquids, even some that resemble chocolate candy bars.

If you are feeling constipated, most **over-the-counter** laxatives—if used correctly—are a harmless and effective way to stimulate a bowel movement. Just be sure to read the label on the package—something you should do before taking any medicine—to learn how much to take and how often to take it.

The label will also alert you to the fact that laxatives can interact with other medications. Laxatives should be taken two or more hours before or after those medications to maintain the effectiveness of those medications. In addition, the label contains warnings about possible reactions that should prompt you to discontinue using the product or consult a physician.

What causes people to misuse laxatives? Often, it's the age-old search for a quick fix. Healthy people may think laxatives are a safe way to get rid of a few unwanted **calories**. Unfortunately, it's not only unsafe but also ineffective.

People who have eating disorders may be much less innocent in their misuse of laxatives. Often, they are so desperate to lose weight or keep from gaining weight that they ignore the warnings and use laxatives as a weapon in their war against calories, taking many times more than the recommended dosage.

KEEPING LAXATIVES A SECRET

Most people like to keep their bathroom habits private. So if a friend doesn't tell you that he or she is taking laxatives, that is probably perfectly normal. They just don't want to talk about something they find embarrassing.

However, people with eating disorders are likely to be secretive about their laxative use because they know they are abusing them and doing something harmful to their body. Occasional laxative use is common, but taking more than the recommended dose is a sign of a problem.

HOW LAXATIVES WORK

To understand how laxatives work, you need a basic understanding of the digestive tract. The journey from food to waste moves from the esophagus to the stomach, from the stomach to the small bowel, and finally from the small bowel to the large bowel—where water is removed from the semiliquid waste—and the rectum.

Laxatives stimulate the large bowel. Before food ever reaches the large bowel, it has to go through the small bowel. The job of the small bowel is to absorb nutrients. The small bowel does its job very efficiently. It absorbs nutrients no matter how quickly food passes through it. The problem for those who use laxatives to control their weight is that laxatives work on the large bowel—after the small bowel has absorbed the calories. Laxatives can cause diarrhea, and consequently, the loss of some water weight, but that's all. They have no effect on real weight loss. This short anatomy lesson is one that people with bulimia who use laxatives as a form of purging have not yet learned.

Q & A

Question: If my sister were taking several laxatives a day, wouldn't I notice it?

Answer: Not necessarily. People with bulimia are usually good at hiding their activities. Besides concealing their supply of laxatives, they are likely to clean the toilet and use air freshener. Some even go so far as to use the shower as a toilet so that all evidence is washed away.

PHYSICAL EFFECTS OF MISUSE

Some people take a laxative every day to increase the frequency of their bowel movements. They quickly discover that with continued use, the body builds a tolerance to the chemicals in the laxative, requiring an increase in dosage to achieve the same effect. So, the more laxatives someone takes, the more laxatives he or she seems to need. Abuse, and the physical results of abuse, can happen quickly.

Diarrhea can be unpleasant, but laxative abuse causes many other physical symptoms as well. When laxatives overstimulate the bowel, the result may be cramps, sometimes very severe ones. Another consequence may be nausea. Frequent wiping after bowel movements may also cause irritation and pain.

Laxatives also cause **dehydration**—a loss of fluids from the body—because they disturb the balance of electrolytes in much the way vomiting does. Electrolytes are minerals in the blood and body fluids that affect how much water is in the body. In mild cases, people who overuse laxatives may fall or faint easily. In serious cases, they may die of dehydration.

People who abuse laxatives do not find it easy to stop taking them. Discontinuing laxatives can result in new problems. Because the large bowel has begun to rely on artificial stimulation, it will not immediately return to normal function. Therefore those who have become dependent on laxatives often experience constipation and bloating when they try to give up laxatives. In extreme cases, the nerve network of the bowel may stop working and surgery may be required to remove part of the bowel.

Fact Or Fiction

Herbal laxatives are safe, because they're sold at the health food store.

The Facts: Health food stores sell herbal laxatives, usually labeled as "dieter's tea" or something similar. Don't be fooled into thinking "herbal" or "natural" means these laxatives are safe. Misused, they cause the same problems as over-the-counter laxatives. The FDA has expressed particular concerns about laxative teas and **supplements** that contain senna, aloe, rhubarb root, buckthorn, cascara, and castor oil. These plant-derived products are not new. Although they have been used to relieve constipation since ancient times, they cause health problems if they are overused. Several herbal substances, including cascara, senna, and castor oil, are also available in over-the-counter laxatives, which the FDA regulates.

PRODUCTS SIMILAR TO LAXATIVES

Laxatives are not the only medication that people with eating disorders use in an attempt to affect their bodily functions. Many also use **diuretics** (some people call them water pills). They are chemicals that cause people to urinate more often than normal. Some pharmacies and health food stores carry over-the-counter diuretics, but most are prescription drugs. They are meant to be used under the supervision of a physician.

Diuretics do not remove calories or fat, but they do result in a loss of water weight. If abused, diuretics often cause dehydration and disrupt body chemicals.

People with eating disorders may also use suppositories (medicines that are inserted in the rectum) to stimulate bowel movement. Unlike laxatives, suppositories work on the small bowel. Like laxatives, the chemicals in these substances do not prevent the absorption of calories or get rid of fat. Enemas are like suppositories but in a different form. Unlike suppositories, which are small solid objects, enemas are liquids that are inserted rectally to move the bowel. All of these products are addictive, expensive, and harmful when abused.

LAXATIVE ABUSE IS DRUG ABUSE

It may sound harsh, but the overuse of laxatives and other FDA-approved, safe, legal, over-the-counter medications is nothing short of drug abuse. Overcoming the habit, much like overcoming any other form of drug abuse, is likely to require time, medical attention, and expert help.

See also: Bulimia; Ethnicity, Genetics, and Eating Disorders; Purging

FURTHER READING
Kirkpatrick, Jim, and Paul Caldwell. *Eating Disorders: Everything You Need to Know.* Rev. ed. Buffalo, N.Y.: Firefly Books, 2004.

■ MEDIA AND EATING DISORDERS

The media consists of all mass communication including newspapers, magazines, direct mail, billboards, radio, television, and the Internet. If you are like most Americans, the many hours you spend with the media shapes what you think of your appearance and how you feel about yourself. That time may even increase the possibility of developing an eating disorder.

Have you ever compared yourself to a celebrity? It's a natural thing to do. Think about the comparison. Did you focus on the celebrity's wit, intelligence, and good nature? Or did you focus on how great the celebrity's body looks or the terrific clothes he or she wears?

Celebrities are expected to look good—it's often part of their job. Many have a staff devoted to helping them maintain their looks. So comparing how you look to how they look is really not a fair comparison—and you probably know that. Still, many people do compare.

The feeling that you don't measure up to your ideal is not a good feeling. That's why study after study has found that people feel negatively about themselves after seeing television shows, music videos, movies, and magazines that portray very thin "ideal women" and muscular "ideal men." Examples of such studies include:

■ "The Role of Television in Adolescent Women's Body Dissatisfaction and Drive for Thinness," a 1996 study published in the International Journal of Eating Disorders, found a correlation between the amount of time teens watch soap operas, movies, and music videos and their degree of dissatisfaction with their own body and their desire to be thin. The more they watch, the greater their dissatisfaction.

■ "The Relationship Between Media Consumption and Eating Disorders," a 1997 study that focused on undergraduates, reached conclusions similar to the 1996 study. Media consumption was positively associated with men striving to be thinner and women feeling dissatisfied with their bodies.

■ "The Effect of Television on Mood and Body Dissatisfaction," a 2002 study, found that teenage girls who watched commercials featuring the "thin is beautiful" ideal felt less confident, more angry, and more dissatisfied with their weight and appearance than those who did not see the ads.

■ A 2002 study, "The Media's Impact on Adolescents' Body Dissatisfaction," examined how teenagers felt after reading magazines and watching music videos, soap operas, and other TV shows. The researchers concluded that teens had negative feelings about their own bodies after seeing images that emphasized the thin ideal. In the study, girls who identified with models and boys who identified with athletes also felt dissatisfied with their own bodies.

■ Yet another 2002 study at the University of Wisconsin, Green Bay, revealed the effects of the media on 10-year-olds. After watching a Britney Spears music video or a clip from the TV show "Friends," the elementary school students expressed dissatisfaction with their own bodies.

DID YOU KNOW?

Comparing American Females to Their TV Counterparts

	American women	Network TV characters
Obese	25%	3%
Underweight	5%	32%

Source: *Health,* April 2002.

■ A study published in the Journal of Research on Adolescence in November 2005 included 136 girls between 11 and 16 years of age in the United Kingdom and found that exposure to magazine models led to lower satisfaction with their own bodies and lower self-esteem. The study also found that the older girls had lower self-esteem than the younger girls.

Fact Or Fiction?

The women who have made headlines because of how great they look have all been very thin.

The Facts: Thin is definitely in fashion today, but it hasn't always been that way. Over several decades, the ideal body has become thinner and thinner. Marilyn Monroe, one of the most well-known beauties of all time, was 5'5" and weighed 135 pounds—she was much curvier than most models and actresses today.

The mass media speaks to "average Americans," but the body images shown in the mass media do not reflect the reality of "average Americans." It's rare to see an **overweight** reporter. Actors spend thousands of hours and dollars (that the average American doesn't have) to stay slim. And even then, close-ups are often enhanced through the use of a body double or digital video effects.

In April 2002, the magazine *Health* checked to see how well the percentage of obese and underweight women appearing as network television characters matched up to the "real life" percentage of obese and underweight American women. Its findings appear in the box on page 113.

TV AND MOVIES

Nielsen Media Research's 2007 statistics found that the average American watches more than four and a half hours of television a day. For the most part, the characters you fall in love with or cheer for on TV and in the movies are not overweight. On the screen, overweight characters get laughs and sometimes pity. Underweight stars play the heroes and the romantic ideals.

To see how TV and movie personalities influence society's image of beauty and style, check the latest fashions and hairstyles. People emulate celebrities or try to. When they can't live up to their ideal—and most people can't—that's when problems often start.

MUSIC AND VIDEOS

Today, eight out of 10 young people will listen to music, according to results of a survey released by The Kaiser Family Foundation in 2005. After surveying more than 2,000 young people, ages eight to 18, the foundation reported that its respondents spent an average of 1 hour 44 minutes listening to music (not including music videos). Teens between 15 and 18 years old spent even more time—2 hours and 24 minutes a day.

Some teens spend as much time listening to music, and maybe even a little more, than they do watching TV. The kind of music they listen to, especially if the songs contain angry lyrics or lyrics that objectify women, can affect how they feel about themselves and other teenagers.

The way women are portrayed in music videos can be as influential, or even more so, than movies and other forms of television. Male musicians often use attractive, sexy, thin women as "accessories" in their videos—the women are there to make the musicians look good. Female musicians typically wear revealing clothing. Their bodies get as much attention as their music, if not more. So, watching music videos is one more reason many adolescents have a distorted image of what their bodies should look like—and one more reason many feel their bodies just don't measure up.

Fact Or Fiction?

Models are healthy and look great.

The Facts: Being overweight and lazy isn't healthy. Eating too little food or exercising too much is not healthy either. A body runs on caloric energy, and most models don't provide their bodies with the nutrients they need. Many of today's supermodels meet the physical criteria for anorexia, which means they are at least 15 percent below a healthy **body mass index (BMI)**. At 25 to 35 percent below a **healthy weight**, fashion models are anything but the picture of health.

FASHION MODELS AND MANNEQUINS

In the early 1950s, leading fashion magazines began featuring very thin models from France. This marked the beginning of a new definition of feminine beauty and a new desire among women to be thin. By the 1970s, the push to be thinner and thinner had reached epidemic proportions in the United Kingdom, the United States, Canada, and, later, Japan.

In the 1980s, the average fashion model weighed 8 percent less than the average woman. Today, the average model weighs 23 percent less. In direct response to this trend, mannequins have also become thinner. In 1950, the average mannequin had 34-inch hips, which matched the average among women in general. By 1990, the average hip measurement for a mannequin had dropped to 31 inches, while the average woman now had a hip measurement of 37 inches. The gap between fashion and reality is widening. In fact, if today's mannequins were real, their percentage of body fat would be so low that they would probably have lost their ability to menstruate.

ADVERTISING

Advertisers are the engine behind many of the messages people watch, read, and listen to. Money from the sale of advertisements helps pay for television and radio programming, magazines, and other mass media. The influence of advertisers goes beyond ads, jingles, and commercials, however. TV and movie producers make extra money through "product placement" deals. Companies pay to have their products incorporated into scenes. The next time you're watching a movie and you see a Levi's-clad hero slam down a can of Coke, jump into a BMW, and race past a Starbucks on his way to the scene of a crime, think about the power of product placement.

According to an article by Bakari Chavanu in *Rethinking Schools Online* in the winter of 1999, by the time you graduate from high school, you will probably have spent twice as much time watching television as attending school. By the age of 17, you will probably have seen 350,000 television commercials.

In 2002, Kelly Brownell, director of Yale's Center for Eating and Weight Disorders, told reporters that the average American child sees 10,000 food ads on TV each year, and 95 percent of those commercials are for fast foods, soft drinks, candy, or sugar cereals. If you think that may be the reason the United States has a growing number of overweight and obese children, you're not alone. Many experts agree.

Experts also think that many people with eating disorders are confused by the mixed messages they receive from the media. Even as the media links thinness to popularity and sex appeal, it promotes fattening, unhealthy foods. Magazines juxtapose articles on the latest diet and exercise trends with recipes for fattening dishes and tempting food ads. The same is also true of television, movies, and other media.

Advertising may also help explain why eating disorders affect many more women than men. Women's magazines generally have about ten times as many ads and articles promoting weight loss as men's magazines.

One advertiser, Dove, began bucking these trends by commissioning The Real Truth About Beauty study, which was completed in September 2004, and launching its "Campaign for Real Beauty." Dove's global study included 3,200 women, ages 18 to 64, in 10 countries, and was led by Dr. Nancy Etcoff of Harvard and Dr. Susie Orbach of the London School of Economics. They found that almost half the women thought they weighed too much and only 2 percent described themselves as beautiful.

In response, Dove changed the way it advertises, featuring everyday women instead of professional models in its ads. Dove also created a self-esteem fund which pays for programs aimed particularly at young teens.

Q & A

Question: Is there any hope that teen magazines will start to place less of an emphasis on dieting and staying thin?

Answer: In 2002, the editor-in-chief of the popular teen magazine *YM* announced that the magazine will no longer publish articles about dieting. Editor Christina Kelly explained, "The need to be super thin is all consuming for many girls, and eating disorders continue to be a major problem. In the age of airbrushing, waif-like pop stars and models, and the quick-fix approach to weight loss, young women need positive examples about body image. *YM* wants to be the catalyst for a change in the way girls think about themselves and their bodies."

THE INTERNET

In 2005, 74 percent of eight- to 18-year-olds had Internet access at home, according to the Kaiser Family Foundation. About half said they had looked for health information and 38 percent had bought something online.

On the Internet, the traditional lines between advertising and information are blurred. Some of the ads are obviously ads. They pop up or appear as a banner and are labeled as advertisements. Many more ads are embedded in games, quizzes, chats, and stories. Both the informational content and the ads contain all of the potentially troublesome elements that are present in other forms of the media.

Used carefully, the Internet can be a valuable resource for information and support. People with eating disorders often become alienated from friends and family. Through the Internet, they can anonymously find resource centers and online **support groups**. When they're ready for help, the very act of discovering that they are not alone in their struggles can be empowering. Before trusting what you find on the Web, however, learn who is hosting the site and find out about their expertise and experience.

Q & A

Question: How do I know what to trust on the Internet?

Answer: You're right to be wary when it comes to the Internet. While the Web is an incredible resource, trusting whatever you see just because you see it in writing is a natural (and dangerous) inclination. In fact, there are many inaccuracies and misinformation, especially on sites hosted by individuals who aren't experts. To avoid these sites, rely on Web sites hosted by well-known universities (with Web addresses ending in .edu) and government agencies (with Web addresses ending in .gov), such as the National Institutes of Health and the Centers for Disease Control and Prevention. In general, pay attention to when information was posted or updated. If there's no date, beware. Check to make sure the Web site provides sources for data. Have credible experts and institutions contributed their knowledge to the site?

SUBLIMINAL MESSAGES

Subliminal messages are ideas that are conveyed so subtly that you may not be aware of them. Unlike TV programs, magazine articles, and Web sites that send a clear message that "thin is in" by focusing on ways to improve one's body through diet and exercise, most messages in the media are less obvious. When a thin actress plays the romantic lead role in a sitcom and an overweight actress plays her funny but unmarried housekeeper, the subliminal message is that outward appearance matters.

BODY TYPES AND ARTISTIC TECHNIQUES

Today people are surrounded by media images of skinny celebrities and models. So you may be surprised or even shocked to learn that some of the world's most famous paintings show full-figured women. In the 17th century, the nude women painted by artist Peter Paul Rubens had rolls of flesh, dimpled buttocks, rounded stomachs, and curved hips. The term *Rubenesque* is used to describe women who reflect his idea of beauty. Van Rijn Rembrandt, who also painted in the early 1600s, used large women in his work as well, although his models became slimmer over time. Pierre Auguste Renoir, a 19th-century artist, is also known for painting nude women with womanly curves. They are not as fleshy as Ruben's nudes, but there is not a bone in sight.

TEENS SPEAK

A Lesson on the Media

This is a story about a teacher who opened up my eyes. When Ms. Alvarez told us we were going to be studying the media, I was excited. I figured we'd be watching TV for homework. Cool.

As it turned out, we did watch a lot of TV, and that was fun, but it was also disturbing. Wow! There was a lot I hadn't realized about what I was watching.

This is how a typical class would go. She had started out by showing us something on TV—either a commercial or a clip (a part of a program). Then, she'd ask us to write five things we noticed in the clip. We were looking specifically for two things—what the clip made us want and how the clip made us feel about ourselves. Then she'd turn the sound off and show us the clip again. We would write more observations. Then she had us just listen to what was said without seeing the video, and we'd write our thoughts again.

It took a while for the first class discussion to really get going. I know I didn't want to say what I was feeling in front of everyone. I wasn't about to admit that I would have traded my entire wardrobe to be able to look like the star of the show. Not that I'm fat or anything, but I don't have her perfect body, that's for sure. And when the conversation got going and the guys started talking, it was clear that if I'd had her looks, I could've been dating any guy in the class.

Okay, so that wasn't exactly earth-shattering. But the surprises came when our teacher talked about the observations we handed in—things we wrote but did not say publicly. It turned out that just about every girl in the class felt the way I did—envious of the "perfect body" we'd seen on screen and pretty negative about how our own bodies look. Most of my friends have great bodies, and I was surprised they didn't think they were good enough.

As the unit went on, we saw how the media emphasizes physical beauty and can influence what we think is hip just by adding good music and a popular celebrity.

GETTING PERSPECTIVE ON THE MEDIA

While the media is overwhelmingly centered on the notion that "thin is in," not everyone accepts that idea. "Plus-size" fashion models pose in all kinds of clothing and project confidence in their bodies. Numerous fashion designers and retailers offer stylish clothes in large sizes. Some magazines focus on the beauty that comes from being healthy and self-confident. Those examples are still the minority, though, while the "thin is in" message is nearly inescapable.

See also: Eating Disorders, Causes of; Peer Pressure; Internet and Eating Disorders, The

FURTHER READING

Levenkron, Steven. *Anatomy of Anorexia.* New York: Lion's Crown, 2000.

Mundell, E. J. "Sitcoms, Videos Make Even Fifth-Graders Feel Fat." Reuters Health. August 26, 2002.

Wykes, Maggie, and Barrie Gunter. *The Media and Body Image: If Looks Could Kill.* Thousand Oaks, Calif.: SAGE, 2005.

■ MORBIDITY AND MORTALITY

Morbidity refers to the harmful effects of a disease and mortality to the deadliness of the disease. If the mortality rate associated with a disease rises, it means that more people are now dying from that disease. As health professionals try to place various diseases into perspective, they discuss morbidity and mortality rates. Eating disorders have the highest mortality rates of any mental illness.

At one time, eating disorders were thought to be the domain of young, Caucasian girls. Today, experts know that they can affect all ages, ethnicities, and genders. What they don't know is morbidity—to what degree the disorder occurs within specific populations. Estimates of how many people in the United States have an eating disorder range from five to ten million, according to the National Institute for Mental Health, the National Eating Disorders Association, the Eating Disorders Coalition, and the National Association of Anorexia Nervosa and Associated Disorders. It's much easier to report on the number of people who have eating disorders than to figure out how many go undiagnosed, but in 1999, the *New England Journal of Medicine* reported that more than half of all people with eating disorders are not diagnosed. Without a diagnosis, there can be no treatment.

And in a study published in *Biological Psychiatry* in 2007 based on the National Comorbidity Survey Replication, researchers talked to thousands of people in the United States who said they'd had eating disorders and found that less than 45 percent of them had sought treatment for those eating disorders. The longer an eating disorder continues without treatment, the more likely it is to result in death.

RATES OF ILLNESS AND DEATH

Anorexia, an eating disorder in which people deny themselves food, is relatively common. Adolescents and young women, the population most affected by anorexia, have a 0.5 to 1 percent risk of developing the eating disorder, according to two physicians—Sarah Pritts and Jeffrey Susman of the University of Cincinnati's College of Medicine. One percent may seem like a small number, but if you consider that 1 in every 100 girls is likely to develop anorexia, the number begins to sound more significant.

Pritts and Susman found that about 4 to 10 percent of those who develop anorexia will die from it. Many of those deaths occur because of **organ failure** or other health problems caused by insufficient nutrition. The high **suicide** rate among people with anorexia may help explain why the mortality rate is so high. To put these statistics in perspective, a 1995 study published in the *American Journal of Psychiatry* found that young women aged 15 to 24 with anorexia are 12 times more likely to die at their age than other young women, and their suicide rate is 75 percent higher. A 2004 study published in the *International Journal of Eating Disorders* looked at health statistics around the world and found suicide to be a major—and underestimated—cause of death among people suffering from anorexia.

The longer a person has had the eating disorder, the more likely he or she is to die from it. According to guidelines published in 2000 by the American Psychiatric Association, anyone who has had anorexia for five years has about a 5 percent chance of dying from the disorder. Someone who has had anorexia for 20 years or more has about a 20 percent of dying from it—a dramatic increase that underscores the importance of diagnosing eating disorders as soon as possible.

Researchers at University of British Columbia analyzed 10 million death records posted in the United States from 1986 to 1990. They found a surprisingly high incidence of mortality among older people with anorexia. More than 78 percent of the deaths that involved anorexia nervosa occurred among people who were more than 45 years of age.

Bulimia and binge-eating disorder are both believed to be more common than anorexia, but not as deadly. A large-scale national survey published in *Biological Psychiatry* in February 2007, using National Institute of Mental Health data from its National Comorbidity Survey Replication, found that while 0.9 percent of women and 0.3 percent of men reported having anorexia, 1.5 percent of women and 0.5 percent of men reported being bulimic, and 3.5 percent of women and 2 percent of men said they had experienced binge-eating disorder during their lifetimes. There are no long-term studies on the mortality rates connected to bulimia or binge-eating disorder yet.

Mortality rates decrease significantly among people who receive treatment for their eating disorder. Anorexia Nervosa and Related Disorders, Inc., estimates that 2 to 3 percent of those who are treated for an eating disorder will die eventually from it, but the mortality rate goes as high as 20 percent for people who have eating disorders but have not received treatment.

POPULATIONS MOST AFFECTED

Today, medical professionals know that eating disorders are not restricted to young, Caucasian girls. However, the American Academy of Family Physicians (AAFP) and other experts note that those young women remain the population that is most affected by such disorders. In fact, a woman's risk of getting an eating disorder is three times higher than a man's risk, and the median age for getting an eating disorder is between 18 and 21 years, according to the latest information from AAFP, released in January 2008.

ANAD reports that in the United States, Latin Americans are as likely as Caucasian women to have an eating disorder and that the incidence among African Americans (particularly in regard to bulimia and laxative abuse) is higher than previously thought.

Researchers at ANAD and other experts in eating disorders note that people who participate in sports and activities in which a small, thin body is emphasized are more likely to develop eating disorders than others. Dancers, ice skaters, gymnasts, runners, swimmers, wrestlers, jockeys, and models fall into that category.

The results of a 10-year study conducted by ANAD reveal that 86 percent of those who reported eating disorders say they began before the age of 20. About 10 percent of those eating disorders started before the age of 10. ANAD also looked at the duration of eating disorders and found that for 30 percent of those surveyed, their disorder lasted between one and five years; 32 percent battled the disorder for six to 10 years; and 16 percent suffered for 11 to 15 years. Only 50 percent of the people they studied claimed to be cured.

COMORBIDITY

Comorbidity is the appearance of two or more diseases or disorders at the same time. Comorbidity does not mean that one disorder causes the other. It means that in many cases, people with one disorder also have another. The more doctors know about the comorbidity of various medical problems, the more likely they are to provide patients with thorough examinations and accurate diagnoses.

In the study "Psychiatric Comorbidities of Female Inpatients with Eating Disorders," published in *Psychosomatic Medicine* in 2006, researchers studied nearly 2,500 female eating disorder patients and found that 94 percent of them had mood disorders, primarily depression. Fifty-six percent of the patients had anxiety disorders, such as **obsessive-compulsive disorder**, and 22 percent of them were substance abusers. Researchers called these comorbidity rates "extremely high."

Another study, "Comorbidity of Anxiety Disorders with Anorexia and Bulimia Nervosa," published in 2004 in the *American Journal of Psychiatry*, included a group of more than 500 patients and documented an even higher rate of anxiety disorders—about two-thirds. The most common anxiety disorders among these patients were obsessive-compulsive disorder and social phobia.

One of the newest areas of comorbidity being researched is an association between attention-deficit/hyperactivity disorder (ADHD) and eating disorders. In 2007 and 2008, researchers at Harvard and Vanderbilt released separate studies showing that girls with ADHD seem to have a greater chance of getting eating disorders.

EATING DISORDERS IN THE FUTURE

Accurately determining rates of mortality and morbidity require long-term studies. In that sense, eating disorders as a field for research is still relatively young, particularly when it comes to research related to bulimia and to males with eating disorders. As researchers continue to gather data on eating disorders, they may be able to shed more light on the prevalence and deadliness of various eating disorders. Perhaps, as awareness and understanding of eating disorders increases, the mortality rates will drop.

See also: Anorexia; Binge-Eating Disorder; Bulimia; Treatment

FURTHER READING
Yancey, Diane. *Eating Disorders.* Brookfield, Conn.: Twenty-first Century Books, 1999.

■ NUTRITION AND NUTRITIONAL DEFICIENCIES

Nutrition is the process of taking in and utilizing food. It is a three-step process that gives the body the nutrients it needs. First, you eat or drink food. Second, your body breaks the food down into nutrients. Third, the nutrients travel through the bloodstream to various parts of the body where they are used to sustain life. Nutritional deficiencies are the lack of nutrients needed by your body.

Habits can be hard to break. So if you establish healthy eating habits at a young age, you'll reap the benefits all of your life. On the other hand, if you decide you've got plenty of time to worry about your health and put off the worrying until well into adulthood, you will find it difficult to break unhealthy eating habits.

HEALTHY EATING HABITS

What will you gain by developing healthy eating habits? According to the Centers for Disease Control and Prevention (CDC), eating right

- helps you grow, develop, and do well in school;
- prevents childhood health problems, including obesity, eating disorders, dental problems, and **anemia** (iron deficiency); and
- may help prevent health problems later in life, including heart disease, cancer, and stroke—the three leading causes of death.

The U.S. Department of Agriculture (USDA) and the U.S. Department of Health and Human Services publish dietary guidelines that suggest Americans eat:

- a variety of grains daily, especially whole grains;
- a variety of fruits and vegetables daily;
- a diet that is low in **saturated fat** and **cholesterol** and moderate in total fat;

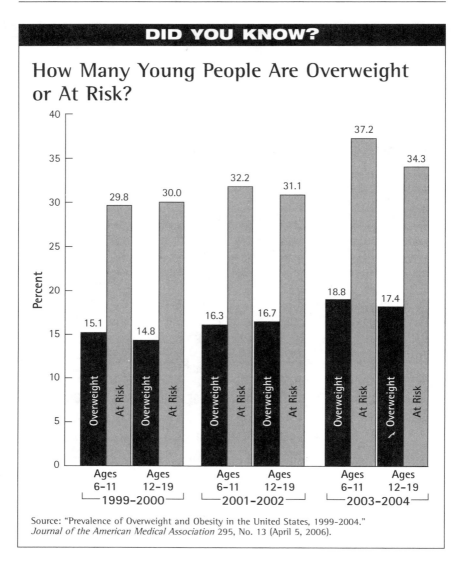

DID YOU KNOW?

How Many Young People Are Overweight or At Risk?

Source: "Prevalence of Overweight and Obesity in the United States, 1999-2004." *Journal of the American Medical Association* 295, No. 13 (April 5, 2006).

■ foods and beverages that contain less sugars; and

■ foods and beverages that contain less salt.

POOR EATING HABITS

Eating unhealthy foods may seem easier or more fun than eating right, but there are consequences. The CDC warns:

- Hungry children are more likely to have behavioral, emotional, and academic problems at school.

- Poor eating habits and inactivity are the root causes of weight problems and obesity. The percentage of young people who are **overweight** has almost doubled in the past 20 years.

- Eating disorders such as anorexia and bulimia—which can cause severe health problems and even death—are increasingly common among young people.

- Nutritional deficiencies in the diet and inactivity cause at least 300,000 deaths among U.S. adults each year.

The percentage of overweight young people has been rising sharply for decades. The CDC reports that from 1980 to 2004, the percentage of overweight six- to 11-year-olds more than doubled, from 7 percent to nearly 19 percent and the percentage of overweight 12- to 19-year-olds more than tripled—from 5 percent to more than 17 percent.

COMMON MISTAKES

Eating too much saturated fat is a common mistake among young people (and older people, for that matter). Saturated fats, which are found in lard, meat, and dairy products, raise cholesterol and increase the risk of heart disease. French fries, donuts, chips, and candy are all loaded with saturated fat. The CDC reports that 72 percent of young people have too much saturated fat in their diet.

Fruits and vegetables are too often ignored. The CDC's 2007 national Youth Risk Behavior Survey found that only about one in five students ate the recommended five or more servings of fruits and vegetables each day. (Fried potatoes, french fries, and potato chips were not considered vegetables by the survey.) Even though females may be likely to order salads, males in the survey were more likely to eat the recommended amount of fruits and vegetables.

The CDC reported in 2000 that one in five high school-aged students regularly skipped breakfast, another common mistake. Some think that avoiding breakfast saves **calories** and time. Yet a breakfast that contains some **protein** and even a little fat along with **complex**

DID YOU KNOW?

How High School Students Eat

	Ate at least 5 servings of fruits and vegetables
Female	19.9%
Male	22.9%

Source: Youth Risk Behavior Survey, 2007.

carbohydrates provides enough energy to last the entire morning. Whole-grain cereal with low-fat or nonfat milk, an egg on toast, or a fruit smoothie made with low-fat or nonfat milk are good choices. Grabbing a danish or a bagel on the way to school is not a good choice. Both are **simple carbohydrates** that will leave most people feeling hungry within an hour or two.

Fact Or Fiction

To be healthy, I need to eliminate fat from my diet.

The Facts: While too much saturated fat can increase your risk of heart disease, some fat actually plays a role in keeping you healthy. Fat insulates your body and helps you absorb certain vitamins. Fat holds your kidneys, heart, and liver in place. Fat also prolongs digestion, making you feel full longer. Unsaturated fats, which are found in vegetable oil, seafood, fish, nuts, seeds, and olives, keep your blood, arteries, and nerves healthy and are important to your growth. When you replace saturated fats with unsaturated fats, you also lower your risk of heart disease.

TEEN NUTRITIONAL NEEDS

At about 10 or 11 years of age, many girls experience a growth spurt that continues until about age 15. Boys have a similar growth spurt. It usually starts around age 12 or 13 and ends at about age 19. These growth spurts place a strain on the body—especially for those who are not eating the right nutrients.

Iron and calcium are especially important during adolescence. All teenagers need iron to support an increasing muscle mass and a larger blood supply. Furthermore, girls lose iron with their monthly period.

Calcium is important for growing bones, and if you don't get enough in your teen years, you risk losing bone mass later. The International Food Information Council Foundation says that teenagers need about 1,300 milligrams of calcium every day, but just two girls in 10 and five boys in 10 ages nine to 19 receive enough, according to a May 2002 article in *U.S. News and World Report*. The average calcium consumption is closer to 800 milligrams a day.

Researchers at the University of Hawaii may have discovered a new incentive for getting the right amount of calcium. In their April 2003 study, they divided 323 girls between ages nine and 14 into two groups. One group of girls ate as usual and consumed on average 881 milligrams of calcium a day. The girls in the second group received more than 1,500 milligrams of calcium a day. The result? The girls in the group that received more calcium weighed less and had lower body fat. In fact, on average, they were 1.9 pounds lighter for every 300 milligrams of calcium they consumed. More studies are needed before these findings can be considered conclusive, but they do show the importance of calcium in the diet.

You can get the recommended amount of calcium by eating three servings of dairy products a day. Consuming shellfish, seeds, calcium-fortified soy products, calcium-fortified juice, broccoli, and green leafy vegetables are other good ways to include more calcium in your diet.

Zinc is another important nutrient during adolescence. It plays a part in sexual development and maturation. Vitamin B_{12} and other B vitamins help ensure healthy nerve and blood cells. Folic acid, which is also called folate, is a B vitamin found in fruits, green leafy vegetables, and fortified cereals. Some birth defects have been attributed to a lack of folic acid during pregnancy.

Getting the right amount of calories is important, too. Severely restricting calories can compromise the body's ability to grow. Teenage girls, active women, most children over age six, and many inactive men need about 2,200 calories per day, according to the USDA. Teenage boys and active men need about 2,800 calories.

BALANCED DIETS

The USDA began providing dietary guidelines in 1894. In 1992, it issued its first Food Guide Pyramid to draw attention to the importance of nutrition and to show Americans how many servings they should eat from each food group. In 1994, the federal government required labels on various food products to show their nutritional content. "Nutrition Facts" labels provide consumers with consistent and easy-to-read information. Thanks to the labels, American consumers have no excuse for not knowing how many calories and how much fat and **carbohydrates** are in their food. It is important to understand that the Nutrition Facts labels are a reference source, not a definitive recommendation. That's because it is based on a 2,000-calorie diet, which may or may not be your recommended calorie intake.

In 2005, the USDA replaced its Food Guide Pyramid, which had been revised several times, with a new approach, called MyPyramid. The MyPyramid symbol is less specific than previous Food Guide Pyramids and is meant to encourage Americans to make healthy food choices. But if you want more specifics, you can get them by going to http://www.mypyramid.gov. The interactive site is full of nutritional advice, but what's really interesting is that you can get recommendations for a **well-balanced diet** specifically tailored for you, taking into account your age, your gender, your height and weight, and your activity level.

The 2005 Dietary Guidelines include the following recommendations. (Remember, the portion sizes are just references based on a 2,000-calorie diet and should be adapted to your particular optimal calorie level.)

- Eat a variety of foods high in nutrients while limiting the intake of saturated fats and **trans fats**, cholesterol, added sugars, salt, and alcohol.
- Follow a balanced eating plan.
- Balance calories consumed with calories expended.
- Eat a variety of fruits and vegetables every day, adding up to two cups of fruit and two and a half cups of vegetables a day.
- Eat a total of six ounces of grains a day, with half coming from whole-grain products.

- Include three cups of low-fat or fat-free milk in your diet daily, or an equivalent amount of calcium sources.
- Limit total fat to 20 to 35 percent of your calories (25 to 35 percent for children and adolescents), with most coming from fish, nuts, vegetable oils, and other unsaturated fats.
- Choose lean, low-fat, or fat-free protein sources.
- Limit your salt intake.

Along with the nutritional advice, both the Dietary Guidelines and MyPyramid encourage balancing what you eat and how much you eat with regular physical activity.

DID YOU KNOW?

The Food Guide Pyramid, 1996

Source: U.S. Department of Agriculture, 1996.

MyPyramid, 2005

Grains	Vegetables	Fruits	Milk	Meats & Beans
Eat at least 3 oz. of whole-grain cereals, rice, or pasta every day.	Eat more dark-green veggies like broccoli, spinach, and other dark, leafy greens.	Eat a variety of fruits.	Go low-fat or fat-free when you choose milk, yogurt, and other milk products.	Choose low-fat or lean meats and poultry.
	Eat more orange vege-tables like car-rots and sweet potatoes.	Choose fresh, frozen, canned, or dried fruit.	If you don't or can't consume milk, choose lactose-free products or other calcium sources.	Bake it, broil it, or grill it.
	Eat more dry beans and peas like pinto beans, kidney beans, and lentils.	Go easy on fruit juices.		Vary your protein routine—choose more fish, beans, peas, nuts, and seeds.

For a 2,000-calorie diet, you need the amounts below from each food group.

- Eat 6 oz. every day.
- Eat 2 ½ cups every day.
- Eat 2 cups every day.
- Get 3 cups every day; for kids aged 2 to 8, it's 2.
- Eat 5 ½ oz. every day.

The new food pyramid, called MyPyramid, symbolizes a personalized approach to healthy eating and physical activity. The wider base stands for foods with little or no solid fats or added sugars; these should be selected more often. The narrower top stands for foods with more added sugars or fats. The more active a person is, the more of these foods can be consumed. In other words, find your balance between food and physical activity.

Source: U. S. Department of Agriculture, April, 2005.

Q & A

Question: What's in a serving?

Answer: According to the Dietary Guidelines, a serving is one ounce of cereal, a half of a cup of pasta or rice, or one slice of bread. A serving is also is one cup of lettuce, a half of a cup of cooked vegetables, one-third to three-fourths of a cup of fruit juice, or a medium-sized apple or grapefruit. Eight ounces of yogurt, one cup of milk, two ounces of processed cheese is each considered a single serving, as is one ounce of lean meat, or one egg, or one tablespoon of peanut butter. Knowing the size of a serving will help you to understand Nutrition Facts labels, but most important is knowing how many servings are healthy for you. That depends on your age, gender, size, and activity level. If you go to http://mypyramid.gov, you can find specific recommendations just for you. You should be eating from all the food groups, and the number of recommended servings will differ for each.

VEGETARIAN DIETS

Some people choose to follow a vegetarian diet because of moral convictions, while many others do so because they think it is a healthier way to eat. Just cutting out meat, however, does not make you healthy. For example, consider two people ordering lunch at a Mexican restaurant. Whose choices are healthier: The vegetarian who chooses chips and guacamole, refried beans, and cheese quesadillas, or the non-vegetarian who orders beef fajitas? Fajitas are generally made with lean cuts of beef that are grilled, which keeps the fat content relatively low, while every item the vegetarian chose is laden with fat and calories.

The moral is that vegetarians have to be as conscious of nutrition as nonvegetarians. Teenage vegetarians, especially **vegans** (vegetarians who avoid all dairy products), have to be particularly careful to get enough protein, calcium, iron, zinc, and vitamin B_{12} in their diets.

Soy products, beans, peas, and nuts are good sources of protein. Vegetarians who eat dairy can also get protein from eggs and dairy products. For those who don't eat dairy foods, calcium can be found in green leafy vegetables, broccoli, and calcium-fortified soy products and juices. You need vitamin D to help your body process the calcium, so check the labels on fortified products to make sure that vitamin D is included.

Iron is found in beans and nuts, dried fruits, and dark green vegetables. The iron is absorbed best if eaten with foods that are high in vitamin C—foods such as citrus fruits, tomatoes, and potatoes. Yogurt, tofu, whole grains, peas, nuts, and beans are good sources of zinc. Milk, fortified soy milk, fortified cereal, miso, tempeh, and sea vegetables (such as nori, which is used to wrap sushi) are all high in vitamin B_{12}. Sea vegetables are sold at natural food stores and Asian groceries.

TEENS SPEAK

How I Became an Independent Eater

It isn't always easy being a vegetarian, especially when you live with meat-eating parents and siblings. I should know. I've been doing it for two years now. My decision to become a vegetarian wasn't an easy one, because I liked the taste of meat. I did it for many reasons: I care about animals; one of my best friends was doing it; I believe I will live a longer and healthier life as a vegetarian; and it is a way to express my individuality. I had lots of reasons, but really no clue as to what it would be like.

When I told my parents I had decided to become a vegetarian, they were surprised. They weren't willing to go to a huge amount of effort to accommodate me. At first, my mother would make her normal meals and I would just eat more of the vegetables and bread and none of the meat. But after a while, we sat down and talked about what I was eating and I realized I wasn't really being all that healthy. Just avoiding meat wasn't enough.

My mother made a deal with me. If I was going to be a vegetarian, I had to read up on it and work to make sure I was following a healthy diet. And I had to learn to cook. In return, my family would agree to eat the veggie meals I cooked at least a couple times a week. On the days when I didn't cook for the family, I had to make sure I could adapt my mother's dinner into something that would include all the nutrients I needed.

It was simple really. I could easily substitute my mother's meaty main dish with a peanut butter sandwich, beans, scrambled eggs, or cheese. And I have become a pretty good cook. I am also much more aware of what it takes to be a healthy eater. Aside from the fact that I knew I shouldn't eat too much fat or too many sweets, I never really paid a lot of attention to the balance of foods that are important. Now, I don't just look for new vegetarian recipes, I look for low-fat vegetarian recipes that include whole grains and lots of different types of vegetables. Some of my recipes have even become family favorites. In the end, I think my little independent streak is going to make my whole family healthier.

KNOWING NUTRITION PAYS OFF

Whether you follow a vegetarian diet or eat meat, knowing your nutritional needs now and making an effort to meet those needs is something that is likely to improve your overall health, well-being, and longevity. As you get older, your body and your lifestyle will change, and you'll need to adjust your nutrition goals accordingly.

See also: Caloric Intake and Expenditures; Fad Diets; Obesity; Weight Control

FURTHER READING

Kaehler, Kathy. *Teenage Fitness: Get Fit, Look Good and Feel Great!* New York: HarperResource, 2001.

Shanley, Ellen, and Colleen Thompson. *Fueling the Teen Machine.* Boulder, Co.: Bull Publishing, 2001.

U.S. Department of Agriculture. MyPyramid.gov. "Steps to a Healthier You." URL: http://mypyramid.gov.

■ OBESITY

The condition of having a **body mass index (BMI)** of 30 or above. Obesity is more than just a number on the body mass index, though. It is more than extra weight or even body fat. It is a complex chronic disease and, like anorexia and bulimia, it is caused by a combination of social, behavioral, cultural, physiological, metabolic, and genetic factors.

Experts use the body mass index to measure body fat content. If a person's BMI is between 18.5 and 25, he or she is in a **healthy weight range**. Those with a BMI between 25 and 30 are considered **overweight**. If one's BMI is 30 or above, he or she is considered obese.

The body mass index isn't perfect. Very muscular people can have BMIs that would classify them as overweight or even obese, but in their case it's muscle, not fat, that pushes them up the scale. A BMI can also underestimate the amount of fat in older people or others who have lost muscle. When people have very little muscle, their BMI may be low even though they have an unhealthy amount of fat. Children and teens should calculate their BMIs based on BMI-for-age growth charts, which account for the differences in fat that is normal for boys and girls at different ages.

OBESITY AS A GROWING PROBLEM

In 2006, Americans were twice as likely to be obese as they were in 1980. In its 2005–2006 National Health and Nutrition Examination Survey, the Centers for Disease Control and Prevention (CDC) found that over 72 million Americans—more than one-third—over the age of 20 were obese. In looking at the distribution of BMIs among those surveyed in the 1976–1980 survey and the 2005–2006 survey, the CDC found that the entire adult population had become heavier, and those with the highest BMIs had gained the most.

The statistics on children and teens (six to 19 years old) reported by the CDC are even more dramatic. Between 1980 and 2004, the number of overweight children and teens had tripled to more than 17 percent, putting more than 12 and a half million young people at risk of diabetes, hypertension, and low self-esteem. Teen girls who are obese may also be at risk of developing depression or anxiety as adults, according to a study published in late 2007. The study followed nearly 800 children and teens for 20 years.

Fact Or Fiction

Being overweight isn't a "life or death" kind of problem.

The Facts: In a report published in 2005, the CDC found that 112,000 obese Americans died prematurely in 2000. Obesity is also an expensive problem, adding up more than $117 billion in medical and related costs in 2000, according to the CDC.

HEALTH PROBLEMS

A long list of medical problems are associated with weight gain, including heart disease, **stroke, high blood pressure**, diabetes, gallbladder disease, and gout (pain in the joints). Being overweight or obese may place people at risk of sleep apnea, a sleep disorder in which a person's breathing stops in intervals that may last from 10 seconds to a minute or longer. The extra weight carried by people who are obese can literally wear away their joints. They may develop osteoarthritis, a degenerative joint disease that causes inflammation, swelling, pain, and stiffness.

Mounting evidence indicates a relationship between obesity and cancer. After following more than 900,000 people throughout the nation for 16 years, the American Cancer Society in 2003 reported that obesity accounts for 14 percent of cancers in men and 20 percent of cancers in women. Researchers concluded that being overweight increases the risk of virtually every form of cancer. They have also discovered that how overweight an individual is affects the size of his or her risk. Men with a BMI of 40 or higher were 52 percent more likely to die from cancer than those with a lower BMI and women with a BMI of 40 or higher were 62 percent more likely to die from cancer.

Researchers are still examining these and other links between obesity and cancer. They know, for example, that if a person has a large amount of fat tissue, his or her body produces too much estrogen and other **hormones** that affect how the cells in the body work. Those hormones may play a role in breast and other cancers related to the **endocrine system**.

Researchers have also learned that obesity can cause gastroesophageal reflux, a disease that causes heartburn when acid from the stomach flows up into the throat. Having gastroesophageal reflux tends to increase the risk of developing cancer in the esophagus.

In addition, the American Cancer Society found that people who are obese do not go to the doctor as often as people whose weight

DID YOU KNOW?

BMI Distribution Among Adults Aged 20–74 Years: 1980 and 2006

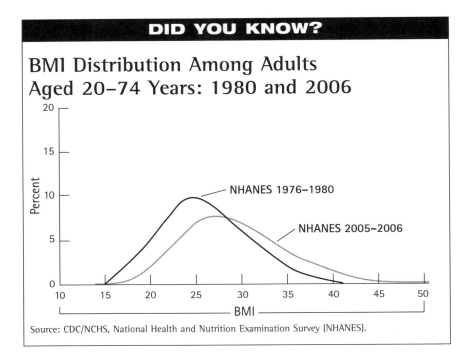

NHANES 1976–1980

NHANES 2005–2006

Source: CDC/NCHS, National Health and Nutrition Examination Survey (NHANES).

is in a healthier range. They may be embarrassed by their weight or find it difficult to travel. Therefore, those who develop cancer are not as likely to be diagnosed early. Detecting cancer is also more difficult because excess tissues may hide the cancer. Even treating cancer is more complicated, because fat absorbs the drugs used in chemotherapy.

The connection between cancer and obesity is serious enough that the American Cancer Society sponsors the "Great American Eat Right Challenge" to increase awareness and encourage Americans to eat healthy and exercise. They also encourage you to include foods that are rich in **antioxidants**, which lowers the risk of some kinds of cancer.

David Satcher, when he was surgeon general in 2001, issued a "call to action" to prevent and decrease obesity, which many believe has become a public health epidemic. The strategies in his call to action included making physical education a requirement at all grade levels and providing healthier food in school cafeterias.

In 2007 the U.S. Department of Health and Human Services launched an initiative to prevent children from becoming overweight and obese, in hopes that establishing healthy habits at an early age will help in the fight to lessen obesity throughout America.

BODY FAT

Gender affects how much body fat one has. Girls start out with 10 to 15 percent more body fat than boys. After puberty, the percentage increases; girls have 20 to 30 percent more body fat than boys. A boy's growth spurt is usually the result of an increase in muscle and lean tissue, while a girl's growth spurt is usually due

DID YOU KNOW?

The Body Mass Index

BMI (Body Mass Index)

Source: U.S. Department of Health and Human Services, 2000.

to an increase in fat tissue. The extra fat is a normal part of sexual development.

Where a person carries his or her body fat can also make a difference. Fat in the abdominal area seems to be more dangerous than carrying extra fat in the thighs or hips. Health experts say that men with a waist that is more than 40 inches and women with a waist of 35 inches or more are at risk of serious health problems.

Another way to assess your health risk is to calculate the ratio of fat around your waist to the fat around your hips and thighs. Most people know how to measure their waist. If you aren't sure where to measure, try about two inches above your belly button. The next measurement should be around the widest part of your hips and thighs. It helps to stand in front of a mirror to be sure you're getting accurate measurements. Then divide the waist measurement by the hip/thigh measurement. Health risks are believed to occur among men with a ratio of 1.0 or more and women with a ratio of 0.8 or more.

Jules Hirsch and Rudolph Liebel, researchers at Rockefeller University, found that fat cells in the abdomen react differently to hormones in the body. They are especially interested in the fact that fat cells seem to be more resistant to **insulin,** a hormone that helps the body convert sugar into energy. As a result, the body produces more insulin. Their findings may explain the connection between abdominal fat and an increased risk of diabetes and heart disease. Since more men than women carry extra abdominal fat, their findings may also help explain why men are more prone to heart disease than women.

People who go on and off diets frequently have a tendency to put on more abdominal fat. That's one reason to think twice before going on a fad diet.

Q & A

Question: Is there such thing as a "fat gene?"

Answer: Both human and animal studies have shown that genetics can play a role in being overweight or obese. At least several dozen genes are involved in obesity, according to the American Dietetic Association (ADA). In 1994, scientists discovered a new hormone that is produced by fat cells and affects how the body regulates weight and feelings of fullness. The hormone is called leptin. Those who are obese tend to have "an excess of circulating leptin in direct proportion to their body mass index," according to the ADA. People with anorexia typically have very low levels of leptin.

NORMAL VS. OVERWEIGHT

What does it mean to have a BMI in the overweight or obese range? Experts have a variety of answers. The dietary guidelines established by the Department of Agriculture suggest that even those who are mildly overweight should try to reduce their weight. The National Heart, Lung and Blood Institute (NHLBI) guidelines recommend losing weight only if you also have two other health **risk factors**. The NHLBI views the following as risk factors:

- a personal or family history of heart disease;
- being a male over the age of 45;
- being a postmenopausal female;
- a history of cigarette smoking;
- a sedentary lifestyle;
- high blood pressure;
- high LDL **cholesterol**;
- low HDL cholesterol;
- high triglycerides; and
- diabetes.

The more risk factors people have, the more benefit they are likely to gain from bringing their weight down to a healthier level.

The Department of Agriculture and the National Heart, Lung and Blood Institute agrees that reducing one's weight by just 10 percent can improve health. Although many overweight people, once motivated to lose weight, set loftier goals, it's important to recognize that a 10 percent drop in weight is a significant achievement.

Assessing obesity

In diagnosing and treating obesity, health-care professionals make assessments (systematic evaluations). A medical assessment is likely to include a variety of measurements, including height, weight, and waist size. The examination tries to rule out organic causes of weight gain, review health risks, and pinpoint health conditions that could affect or be affected by a weight loss.

A psychological assessment screens for mental health disorders that may prevent or complicate successful weight loss efforts. A mental-health professional is likely to look for signs of depression, post-traumatic stress disorder, anxiety, bipolar disorder, addictions, binge-eating disorder, and bulimia.

A nutritional assessment focuses on current eating patterns, weight gains, and dieting history. It also lists all supplements or diet products that the individual may be taking and how ready and willing he or she is to lose weight. Like the psychological assessment, the nutritional assessment may identify factors that might interfere with a successful weight loss—such as physical limitations, time constraints, and knowledge of nutrition.

Finally, a health-care professional will assess one's level of physical activity and motivation to increase that level. When someone is motivated to exercise and finds activities that he or she enjoys, weight loss and improved health is faster and easier to achieve.

Overweight teens

According to the 2005 National Youth Risk Behavior Survey, 15.7 percent of American students were at risk of becoming overweight and 13.1 percent were overweight. Male students were more likely to

DID YOU KNOW?

Students Trying to Lose Weight

	Obese	Overweight	Thought they were overweight	Were trying to lose weight
Female	9.6%	15.1%	34.5%	60.3%
Male	16.3%	16.4%	24.2%	30.4%

Source: Youth Risk Behavior Survey, 2007.

be overweight or at greater risk of becoming overweight than female students. African American and Latino students were more likely to be overweight or at risk of becoming overweight than Caucasian students.

The survey also found that students' perceptions of their weight didn't always match reality. Nationwide, 31.5 percent of all students thought they were overweight, with female students (38.1 percent) significantly more likely to consider themselves overweight than male students (25.1 percent).

High school students aren't nearly as overweight as they think, according to the 2005 Youth Risk Behavior Survey. The survey considered students at or above the 85th percentile but less than the 95th percentile on the BMI chart as "at risk for becoming overweight." Students who were above the 95th percentile on the BMI chart were considered "overweight."

TEENS SPEAK

My Life with 20 Extra Pounds

I hear the whispered comments and my face burns. Then someone does something mean at lunch like grabbing my chips and saying, "You don't need those." I have to go searching through my purse as if I'll die if I don't find a pen right then, just so no one sees the tears in my eyes.

If you didn't know me, you'd read this and assume I'm a big fat slob who sits alone in the cafeteria with no friends and no social life. Actually, you're wrong. I'm not the most popular girl in school, but I have a large group of friends and a small group of close friends and really shouldn't complain at all about my high school experience.

The whispered comments that make my face burn are not meant in a mean way. The comments come from friends who feel bad when something comes up that makes it obvious that I'm 20 pounds overweight and they aren't. Like when our service club plans a car wash and I'm the only one not wearing a bikini top. The "mean" comments about the chips are just people joking, the same way they joke around with the skinny girls. They just want some chips, but I'm a little oversensitive about comments like those.

I'd love nothing more than to lose weight, but I just don't have the will power. I know I really don't need those chips. My mom does the grocery shopping and when there's junk food around the house, I have a hard time not eating it.

Last week I went to the doctor for a physical. I was nervous and definitely expecting a lecture about my weight. To my surprise, the doctor seemed to understand how I felt. She said that I would be healthier if I lost weight and gave me a plan for increasing my exercise and changing my eating habits. She told me not to go on a diet, but just change my habits. She said that all I had to do was lose 10 pounds to be in a healthy weight range.

When I walked out of the office, my mother was waiting for me. At home, we talked about the things the doctor told me about what to eat and what not to eat. My mother promised to try and follow the guidelines the doctor had laid out. As it turns out, she'd been told the same thing during her physical.

TAKING OBESITY SERIOUSLY

Statistics on obesity should be taken seriously. The real problem with being obese isn't that one can't wear the latest fashions or has difficulty fitting into a seat on an airplane. The real problem is that obesity is unhealthy. In fact, being obese can be deadly.

See also: Caloric Intake and Expenditures; Exercise; Nutrition and Nutritional Deficiencies; Stress and Eating Habits; Weight Control

FURTHER READING
Gay, Kathlyn. *Am I Fat?* Berkeley Heights, N.J.: Enslow Publishers, 2006.
Kaehler, Kathy. *Teenage Fitness: Get Fit, Look Good and Feel Great!* New York: HarperResource, 2001.

■ OVEREATING

See: Eating Disorders, Causes of; Obesity

■ PEER PRESSURE

The strong influence that one's peers have on attitudes and behavior. A peer is a person who is one's equal in age and social standing. Everyone experiences peer pressure, but it tends to be at its strongest during adolescence.

Peer pressure can be outspoken and direct, as it is when someone looks at your new jeans and says, "Those are so uncool." Peer pressure can also be subtle and indirect, as it is when you notice that everyone on the tennis team wears the same brand of tennis shoes. No one said you couldn't pick out another brand, but if you know everyone else chose a particular brand, you may feel that you should wear the same shoes everyone else is wearing.

Teenagers are vulnerable to peer pressure because they are still figuring out who they are. If people your age make fun of you or say bad things about you, it can send your self-esteem plummeting. As your self-esteem drops, your risk of developing an eating disorder may increase.

Praise also has an effect. If your peers compliment you on the way you look, you may center your self-image on your appearance, which also increases the risk of an eating disorder. Because self-esteem is fragile during adolescence, teens often have an intense desire to be part of a crowd. Teens may go along with what everyone else is doing, even if it involves making bad choices about drugs, cigarettes, alcohol, or sex.

PEER NORMS

Peer norms are the common expectations and behaviors accepted by other people your age. Peer norms are not necessarily the way you *should* act, but the way most people your age *do* act. If all the girls you sit with in the cafeteria make it a habit to skip lunch, then skipping lunch becomes the norm. Sometimes, following the norm is a good thing. Sometimes, following the norm can be harmful—for example, when the norm is something dangerous to your health, like smoking.

Every once in a while, people need to consider the norms that they find themselves accepting or rejecting and evaluate whether their decisions are healthy or not. Many people will do what everyone else seems to be doing simply because they don't think about going against the norm. They do what they see other people do. Sometimes people follow the norm because they are afraid of the consequences that may follow if they break the norm. They fear peer pressure.

SOCIAL PRESSURE

Peer pressure is a type of social pressure. Social pressure goes beyond peer pressure to include what is popular in our larger society. For example, many teenagers feel pressure to dress a certain way. Popular styles often mimic the way celebrities dress, even though many of those celebrities are unnaturally (some even dangerously) thin. Those who don't meet that standard may develop a negative perception of themselves. They may also be abused by their peers. People who are **overweight** are often teased, bullied, and alienated. They may be treated as if they were lazy, stupid, or dirty.

Yet, with all the pressure to be thin and fit, teens are just as likely to feel social pressure to eat. Most social activities include food, and many popular restaurants add to the problem by serving huge portions of food. This creates a clear social conflict—the pressure to look thin vying with the pressure to eat. Some girls resolve the conflict by turning dieting into a form of bonding even though it puts them at risk of **malnutrition** and the development of an eating disorder.

Fact Or Fiction?

Looking thin makes you popular.

The Facts: It's actually self-confidence that makes you popular. Consider Oprah Winfrey, one of the richest and most influential women in the world. While her weight has gone up and down, her popularity has grown. The way she looks is secondary to the incredible self-confidence she exudes. While your world may be very different than Oprah Winfrey's world, the rules are similar. The people who are most popular are the people who are sure of themselves—those who tend to set trends rather than just follow them. You may counter this by saying that none of the overweight people you know are popular, but chances are good that they are not only overweight but also lacking in self-confidence.

SUPPORT FROM PEERS

The opposite of peer pressure is support from peers. Just as peer pressure can damage self-esteem, peer support can boost self-esteem, especially when you care deeply about what your peers think of you. Your parents may praise you, but they are your parents. When a friend offers the same compliment, it can be very powerful. Peer support can be as simple as praising a friend for what he or she does instead of for his or her appearance. Peer support also can be as complicated as figuring out a way to help a friend who isn't admitting to what may be an eating disorder.

Supporting a friend with an eating disorder starts with being nonjudgmental. You need to listen when your friend wants to talk, understand when your friend needs time away from you, and figure out social activities that are enjoyable instead of challenging. It takes time to overcome an eating disorder and patience to be a good friend to someone who is struggling through treatment.

Many organizations encourage positive peer influence—Students Against Drunk Driving (SADD), for example. In an effort to prevent eating disorders, the National Eating Disorders Association has created a national peer **support group** called GO GIRLS! (Giving Our Girls Inspiration and Resources for Lasting Self-Esteem). The group describes itself as "high school girls working together to promote responsible advertising and to advocate for positive body images of youth by the media and major retailers." The girls participate in group discussions that are meant to strengthen their own personal self-esteem and body image. They learn that their viewpoints can affect and change society.

RECENT TRENDS IN EATING DISORDERS

Many years ago, eating disorders were not openly discussed or readily diagnosed, and those suffering from eating disorders had a difficult time finding treatment. Some experts didn't even acknowledge that eating disorders were genuine illnesses.

Today, eating disorders are well known, well documented, and well researched. Becoming educated on eating disorders is as easy as stepping into a library or going on the Internet. Yet eating disorders continue to be a problem that affects millions of Americans. The latest research shows that girls, boys, men, women, rich, poor, those living in urban and rural areas, the young, and the elderly are all affected. No one is immune.

Fortunately, the accessibility of treatment and support has expanded dramatically, too, and can be found in specialized clinics, residential programs, hospitals, independent practices, and online. People with eating disorders are treated in a much more sophisticated manner than ever before, involving an array of specialists that deal with the physical, emotional, social and nutritional aspects of the disorder. New **psychopharmacological** drugs, which treat the symptoms of mental illnesses, are being prescribed to help patients overcome eating disorders.

On the negative side, societal norms continue to influence the development of eating disorders. People are even using the Internet to flaunt extreme eating and dieting habits, acting as teachers and cheerleaders for those who have an eating disorder or may be on their way to developing one.

In recent years, the "Westernization" of some nations has led to an increase in eating disorders in other parts of the world. Natives of Asia and the Caribbean who have moved to the United States and Europe are especially at risk. They are confronted by the conflicts that Westerners have long dealt with—the message that thin is beautiful, and the temptation of rich, fattening, easily obtained food backed by expensive advertising campaigns and marketing efforts.

FROM PEER PRESSURE TO SOCIETAL TREND

Peer pressure, which starts on a personal level and at a small scale, can spread and develop into societal trends. Thanks to mass media, trends spread more quickly than ever. When a mainstream trend coincides with peer pressure, it is especially difficult to resist.

See also: Eating Disorders, Causes of; Self-Image

FURTHER READING

Arnold, Carrie. *Next to Nothing: A Firsthand Account of One Teenager's Experience with an Eating Disorder.* New York: Oxford University Press, 2007.

Bryan, Jenny. *Eating Disorders.* Austin, Tx.: Raintree Steck-Vaughn Publishers, 2000.

Normandi, Carol Emery, and Laurelee Roark. *Over It.* Novato, Calif.: New World Library, 2001.

■ PURGING

An attempt to erase the consequences of a **binge** by vomiting, using laxatives or **diuretics**, or even exercising excessively. People with bulimia who binge and then purge on a regular basis may actually feel "cleansed" after purging. But the good feeling doesn't last long, because regular purging is an extremely dangerous thing to do.

Have you ever known someone who was desperate for a quick and easy way to lose weight or to avoid gaining weight? Many people are. They care about their physical appearance and feel they have to be thin to be attractive. Perhaps they work hard to stay thin or perhaps it comes naturally. Either way, they find the thought of being fat repulsive. Yet they are tempted by fattening foods and tasty dishes: the bacon their mother cooks for breakfast, pizza in the cafeteria, fries and milk shakes at a fast-food restaurant on the way home from school, candy and chips in a vending machine.

Temptation is everywhere. Some may give in to it from time to time. Perhaps they find that once they start eating, they can't stop. What happens next? Unfortunately, for a few people, the solution is purging. They find ways to rid their body of all those **calories** and start over. It seems like magic and seems so much easier than avoiding the junk food or dieting.

IDENTIFYING BEHAVIORS

People purge by vomiting, using laxatives or diuretics, fasting, or exercising obsessively. Any one of these behaviors can take a serious toll on the body. People who make themselves vomit often reach a point where they don't have to do anything to vomit but think about it. In fact, in some cases, vomiting becomes an uncontrollable response. People who binge and then vomit may even choose what to eat based on which foods are easiest to bring back up.

Other people use **Ipecac syrup** to make themselves vomit. Ipecac syrup is a thick liquid that many parents keep on hand as a safety precaution. They use it to induce vomiting if their child ingests a poisonous substance. However, when the syrup is abused, it can damage the heart or skeletal muscles. It can even cause sudden death.

Chronic vomiting brings up stomach acid, which can cause serious tooth decay, swollen salivary glands (which resemble a chipmunk's puffed-out cheeks), and the loss of a dangerous amount of potassium. A low potassium level can result in fatal heart problems.

Vomiting can also damage the stomach and kidneys. Stomach pain may become constant.

Abusing laxatives and diuretics also has side effects, including severe cramps, **dehydration** (loss or lack of liquid in the body), and bowel dysfunction. Ironically, laxatives and diuretics are not effective ways of ridding the body of unwanted fat. They simply rid the body of water weight.

Fasting is yet another way of abusing the body. It, too, can lead to dehydration, **lethargy** (lack of energy), light-headedness, and kidney damage. Extreme exercise can also be a form of purging, one that not only causes dehydration but also broken bones, torn ligaments, joint problems, osteoporosis (progressive loss of bone density), muscle damage, and even heart and kidney failure.

It can be hard to determine if a friend or relative is using one or more of these methods to purge. People who purge generally hide what they are doing and lie about it. Moreover, if they're bingeing and purging, they may be maintaining the same weight—making it even harder to detect a problem.

One way to identify someone who purges is by paying attention to everyday actions. People who purge often become so obsessed with when, where, and how to purge that they alienate friends and family and withdraw from everyday activities.

RATES

The National Institute of Mental Health (NIMH) classifies people who binge and purge at least twice a week for three months as bulimic. Bulimia affects men as well as women. A study published in the *American Journal of Psychiatry* in 2001, "Comparisons of Men with Full or Partial Eating Disorders, Men without Eating Disorders, and Women with Eating Disorders in the Community," reports that for every eight to 11 females with bulimia, there is one male with the disorder. The Harvard Eating Disorders Clinic estimates that men account for 10 to 15 percent of the reported cases of bulimia.

From February 2001 to December 2003, NIMH funded a national survey (called the National Comorbidity Survey Replication) in which nearly 3,000 adults were asked about eating disorders. In 2007 an analysis of the data was published in *Biological Psychiatry*, and in it, researchers reported that 1.5 percent of the women and 0.5 percent of the men said they'd had bulimia at some point in their lives. If you do the math, this survey suggests that there may be a higher ratio of men suffering from bulimia than previously reported—approximately three men for every nine women, or 33 percent.

RESPONSES

Anyone who purges or knows someone who does needs to get help as quickly as possible. People who purge often need the help of a team of health-care professionals—a physician to deal with the physical health problems, a **psychotherapist** for emotional problems, and a **nutritionist** to teach healthy eating habits—in overcoming the desire to purge and develop a healthier lifestyle.

Even after treatment, numerous studies indicate that the possibility of a **relapse** is a major concern. They reveal that about 25 percent of patients in **remission** (an absence of binge and purge episodes for at least four weeks) had a relapse in less than three months. After nine months, 51 percent had a relapse. After four years with no symptoms of bulimia, the risk of relapse seems to decline.

TEENS SPEAK

How Purging Took Control over My Life

I had purging down to a science. In fact, my purging routines gave me a sense of power.

I started every day by skipping breakfast. Mom might have worried about that, but I always grabbed something to take with me as I left in a rush for school. I didn't like throwing food away, so I'd give it to one of my guy friends who always seemed to be hungry. At lunch, I ate something small, like a salad, which was pretty much what most girls at school eat. But I couldn't stand having even that small amount of food in my stomach. I was worried about getting fat. Since they are so easy to get rid of, why let those calories hang around? I headed right from the cafeteria to the bathroom. I knew exactly which bathroom to go to, one that was near the gym and usually deserted at lunchtime.

When I first started purging, I used to stick my finger down my throat, but it wasn't long before I could just think about vomiting and throw up. So, my lunchtime bathroom excursion was quick. I always kept sugarless gum in my purse, so my breath would never give me away.

After school, if I came home before anyone else, I usually binged on sweets, bread, chips, leftovers, whatever I could find. I was careful to hide the evidence of each food I ate before moving on to the next. That way, if someone came home, it wasn't obvious how much I had eaten.

My mom used to comment on how lucky I was to be able to eat junk food and stay thin, but she had no idea how much I was eating. Sometimes I even volunteered to do the grocery shopping so that I could get extra food and hide it in my room or behind other stuff in the refrigerator. After the binge, I would feel terrible about myself, but I knew that I could easily erase my actions. I'd go upstairs, vomit, and feel not only relieved but also empowered. After that, I'd exercise, do homework, and then exercise again. I even put folded-up blankets on the floor so that I could run in place in my room late at night without anyone knowing.

Everything was great unless there was an interruption in my routine. A school trip would have spoiled everything, so I pretended I was sick and didn't go. I got out of a family reunion by saying I had to stay home to work on a huge school project. I even started skipping parties and shopping trips where I knew the bathrooms would be too crowded to vomit in private. One day, after lying in order to stay in the safety of my own home, I began to realize that purging was actually controlling me. Yet I wasn't sure I could stop. Finally, I did the hardest thing I've ever had to do. I asked for help.

PURGING: EXTREME BEHAVIOR

Many people don't realize that purging is more than just vomiting. Purging describes several different types of extreme behaviors, all with the goal of getting rid of what someone considers excess calories. The only safe way to make up for eating too much, though, is to follow a reasonable diet plan that cuts calories and increases activity.

See also: Bulimia; Eating Disorders, Symptoms and Diagnosis of; Internet and Eating Disorders, The; Laxative Abuse

FURTHER READING

Kirkpatrick, Jim, and Paul Caldwell. *Eating Disorders: Everything You Need to Know.* Buffalo, N.Y.: Firefly Books, 2001.
Maine, Margo, Ph.D. *Body Wars: Making Peace with Women's Bodies.* Carlsbad, Calif.: Gurze Books, 2000.
Mendelsohn, Susan. *It's Not About the Weight: Attacking Eating Disorders from the Inside Out.* Lincoln, Neb.: iUniverse, 2007.

■ SELF-IMAGE

How one sees oneself, and how one thinks others see him or her. If you were asked to describe your self-image in three words, what words would you choose? Would your description focus on physical attributes—hair, eyes, weight? Would you describe yourself in terms of the things you do—student, sports fan, guitar player? Or would you choose words that highlight aspects of your personality—caring, shy, conscientious?

Many teenagers (and adults) center a large part of their self-image on the way their body looks. The tendency is hard to overcome in a society that places great emphasis on appearance. Ideally, you are developing a balanced self-image, one that includes not only physical attributes but also personality traits, achievements, talents, family identity, and values.

According to the American Psychological Association (APA), good mental health contributes to positive self-image and healthy, rewarding relationships. A negative self-image may be linked to depression, **anxiety**, an eating disorder, or other mental health problems. You may need to resolve that problem before you can develop a positive self-image.

Unfortunately, some parents don't recognize mental health problems in their children, and some teenagers don't admit to them or seek treatment. If anyone you know suffers from such a problem, he or she is not alone. The APA reports that in any given year, one teenager in every five has at least a mild mental health problem.

BODY IMAGE

Your body image is the way you think and feel about your body, its shape, and size. That image includes what you see or think you see in the mirror and how you picture yourself in your mind. It also reflects your feelings about your height, weight, and even the shape of your body. Two people may have the same body shape but very different body images. One woman might look at her hips and thighs and consider them curvy. The other might see herself as flabby or fat.

How you feel as you move about is part of your body image, too. Are you graceful or clumsy? Are you fragile or strong? What you think of your appearance is also an important component of your body image. People who were teased about being overweight as children may always think of themselves as overweight—despite scales, mirrors, and other evidence to the contrary.

Expecting people to feel great about their body at all times isn't realistic, but to lead a healthy, happy life, they need to have a positive body image most of the time. According to the National Eating Disorders Association, to maintain a positive body image, people need to:

- have a realistic perception of their body;
- understand that their physical appearance doesn't say much about their character or their value as a person;
- refuse to spend time worrying about food, weight, and **calories**; and
- feel comfortable and confident in their body.

What, then, are the characteristics of a negative body image? They include:

- a distorted perception of body shape;
- a feeling that other people are attractive, while one's own body shape is a sign of personal failure;
- feelings of shame, self-consciousness, and anxiety about one's body; and
- feeling uncomfortable and awkward in one's body.

People with eating disorders generally have a negative body image. Their self-image is usually so tied up in their body image that everything else gets pushed aside. Those who have bulimia feel they have to take extreme measures, like purging, to be attractive. People with anorexia typically have a distorted body image. They look in the mirror and see fat where others see skin and bones. And those who engage in binge eating often feel so hopeless and depressed about the way they think their body looks that they turn to food for comfort, escape, or fulfillment of a negative self-image.

SOCIAL MESSAGES

There's no question that Americans value thinness. People who are overweight are stereotyped as lazy or sloppy. People who are thin are considered energetic and in control of their lives, whether they are or not. The stereotypes also extend to business, where thin people are generally assumed to have an easier time finding jobs and winning promotions. They are believed to make friends more easily and experience more success than their overweight counterparts. So society's message is clear: Body image is a critical element of self-image.

Society's messages are most obvious in the media. In fact, they are practically inescapable. Even if you managed to avoid the media, you would still be living in a media-saturated society in which your peers and role models are heavily influenced by what they see and read every day. When fashion turns to clingy fabrics and tight, skin-baring styles, society sends yet another message connecting self-image to body-image.

BUILDING ESTEEM

The number of books, tapes, and Web sites devoted to weight loss are probably equal to the number on building **self-esteem**—positive feelings about oneself. Although resources aren't hard to find, it can be difficult to overcome the negative thoughts you may have about yourself and improve your sense of self-worth.

The stakes are high. The Counseling Center for Human Development at the University of South Florida says that people with high self-esteem are happier and more successful in life. People with low self-esteem have trouble setting goals, developing close personal relationships, and feeling that they are in control of their life. The National Institute of Mental Health links low self-esteem with depression.

The Counseling Center for Human Development recommends these strategies for building self-esteem:

- Objectively take stock of your strengths and weaknesses and understand that everyone has both.

- Don't wait for someone else to encourage you. Give yourself encouragement and believe in your ability to do things.

- Set realistic and reachable goals, and take pride in accomplishing them. Setting distant or unreachable goals sets you up for failure or at least for a lack of immediate gratification. Instead of saying, "I will run a marathon," say, "I will run two miles today, and tomorrow I will run a little farther than I did today."

- Explore your talents and be proud of them.

- Don't try to fit in someone else's mold. Be uniquely yourself.

According to the Nemours Center for Children's Health Media, many people experience a drop in self-esteem when they become teenagers— a time of major changes in one's body and one's life. It's also common for self-esteem to drop when people experience other changes that they can't control, such as a divorce in the family, the end of a relationship, or the loss of a job.

Those who have had low self-esteem for some time may not be able to change their mind about how they feel alone. They may need the help of a psychologist (someone who has a doctorate in psychology), a counselor (a person who provides professional help in dealing with difficulties with emotions and relationships), or a **support group** (a group of people with similar problems who try to help each other).

TEENS SPEAK

My Obsession with Being Fat

Since I started middle school, I look in the mirror each day and think the same thing: "You're fat!" Sometimes, the thoughts are angrier: "You're a fat cow." Other times, they are more specific: "You have the flabbiest arms in the whole eighth grade." But it all comes down to those two words: "You're fat!"

My stepfather had no idea I was so hung up on how I looked. If he did, I'm sure he wouldn't have said the things he did. Once, he pointed out that my clothes were getting a little tight and gave me money to go shopping. He was trying to be nice, but I was mortified. I bought baggy clothes and told my parents they were what everyone was wearing. Another time he asked me if I wanted to go jogging with him. I immediately jumped to the conclusion that he thought I needed to burn extra calories. (And I silently agreed, even though I didn't go jogging because that would be admitting I was fat.)

When I was with my friends, things were no better. We'd go shopping at the mall and I would make up excuses not to try on clothes. When I did, I got my own dressing room where I could undress in private. The thought of my friends seeing my flabby thighs was just too terrible.

One day I realized my negative feelings about my body were infringing on my life. It was the day I got a notice at school about soccer tryouts. I'm a very good soccer player. All my friends and family assumed that I would go out for the team. But I was paralyzed by the thought of dressing and showering in open locker rooms. My mother found the crumpled-up notice in my garbage can and asked me what was going on. All my feelings flooded out. Fortunately for me, my mom is a great listener.

My mom did more than listen, she helped me face my feelings and look at my body realistically. She reminded me that I was supposed to be growing out of my clothes and that body changes at my age are part of life. She handed me the notes from my last doctor's appointment, which showed my weight was average for my height and age. She pulled out pictures of herself at my age. My mom even took pictures of me wearing baggy clothes and fitted clothes, so I could see how much less attractive the baggy clothes were. And she reminded me how great it feels to score a goal and to be a part of a team.

Still, I have times when I look in the mirror and think, "You're fat!" Then I remind myself that having a perfect body would take way too much time away from the other things that make up who I am. I pass the mirror thinking how strong and energetic I feel.

THE FRAGILE SELF-IMAGE

A negative self-image can start a cycle that is difficult to end. Consider a teenager who thinks that he will never be as smart as his older, high-achieving brother. The more he dwells on his brother's successes and his own shortcomings, the more he starts to believe he isn't smart enough. He may avoid studying, believing it's a waste of time. His grades slip, confirming his negative self-image.

Anyone who uses a single quality to define himself or herself is bound to have a fragile self-image. The more qualities that are factored into a person's self-image, the better one's chances are of maintaining a positive self-image.

See also: Depression and Weight; Eating Disorders, Causes of; Eating Disorders, Symptoms and Diagnosis of; Media and Eating Disorders; Peer Pressure

FURTHER READING

Beck, Debra, and Maggie Anthony. *My Feet Aren't Ugly! A Girl's Guide to Loving Herself from the Inside Out.* New York: Beaufort Books, 2007.

Bryan, Jenny. *Eating Disorders.* Austin, Tx.: Raintree Steck-Vaughn Publishers, 2000.

Normandi, Carol Emery, and Laurelee Roark. *Over It.* Novato, Calif.: New World Library, 2001.

■ STRESS AND EATING HABITS

An emotionally disruptive or upsetting response to a challenging internal or external influence. Your teacher tells you that if you don't make an A on her final exam, you'll have to go to summer school and retake the class. You're not going to be satisfied unless you break the school freestyle swimming record. You overhear your best friend make a joke at your expense. Your father criticizes you constantly. Stress comes at you every day and along with dealing with unavoidable situations that happen to you, you create your own stress, internally, because of the expectations you have for yourself.

Consider the situation in which you need to make an A on a test to pass a class. You face the immediate situational stress of time management—figuring out how you can get enough studying in when you have other things to do. Worrying about what your summer will be like if you don't get the A and berating yourself for letting your grades get so low in the first place are examples of internal stress coming from pressure you put on yourself.

Stress isn't always bad. The stress of meeting a deadline might also be the push that you need to get something done. The desire to break the school swimming record may be stressful, but excelling in swimming may lead to increased **self-esteem**, a scholarship, or even an athletic career.

Dealing with constant criticism (whether real or imagined) or losing the ability to trust a friend is stressful to anyone, but these things can be especially stressful for teens who struggle to develop self-esteem and are especially sensitive to peer pressure.

Scientists have studied how stress affects eating habits. For both emotional and biological reasons, stress can lead to overeating and obesity. Stress can also cause anxiety, depression, and other psychological conditions that are associated with eating disorders.

Q & A

Question: My family is moving to a different state, so I will be going to a new school next year. I'm excited, but my mother keeps talking about how stressful it is to move. She's concerned that I am keeping my stress inside and should be talking to her about it. But I'm not worried. Should I be?

Answer: Your mother is probably feeling her own stress about the move, and so she expects you to feel that way, too. But it's not the situation that causes stress, it's your reaction to it. Different people react differently to the same situation. For you, moving is exciting. For your mom, it's stressful.

HOW YOUR BODY REACTS TO STRESS

Do you reach for junk food whenever you have a big study session ahead of you? Well, scientists have found a biological explanation for your tendency to eat fattening food when you're under stress.

Your body has a natural desire to be in a state of balance, called **homeostasis.** If you're dehydrated, you feel thirsty and drink. If you expend a lot of energy, you feel hungry and eat. Your body stays in balance. Stress disrupts homeostasis.

When you experience sudden stress—a potential car collision, for example—your body produces a stress hormone called **cortisol,** goes on high alert, and devotes itself to protecting you from danger. The cortisol moves your body's energy resources to where they will best serve you in this state of emergency. More blood flows to your muscles and your metabolism revs up, making energy available to those muscles. Eventually the cortisol reaches your brain and signals the body that it can relax. The immediate danger is over.

When you experience chronic stress—resulting from an ongoing a personality conflict with a teacher, for example—your body's stress response system does not shut off. Your body instead produces more of the stress hormone, cortisol, and you start depleting your body's energy reserves. When energy courses through your body with no outlet, you will feel anxious and uptight.

At this point, some people reach for chocolate cake or some other sugary, fattening treat. Biologically, eating sugary food is a way to replenish the energy being used in the stress process.

"Stress and Eating," an article in the November 2003 issue of *Psychology Today*, describes the research findings of a team from the University of California at San Francisco. The researchers explained that the cortisol, which is busy moving the energy in your body around, takes all those extra calories from the sugary foods right to your abdomen, where they are stored as fat. Abdominal fat is close to your liver and can be turned quickly into energy. The researchers believe the fat then signals the brain that everything is okay and curbs feelings of depression and anxiety.

EMOTIONAL EATING AS A RESPONSE TO STRESS

Weight gain or weight loss can both be warning signs of stress, according to the American Academy of Family Physcians. Some people have trouble eating when they're upset or under stress. Others tend to eat more.

Researchers with the New York Obesity Research Center published a study in 2002 that compared emotional eating among people who were **overweight**, normal weight, and **underweight**. They found that when experiencing negative emotions, the underweight group ate less, and the overweight group ate more.

Studies have shown that adults and children who actively diet or pay attention to their calorie intake (researchers call this "dietary restraint") tend to eat more when they are stressed, while people who do not actively monitor their caloric intake do not eat more under stress. Researchers think that restrained eaters may eat more to distract themselves from the stress they are feeling or because stress lowers the inhibitions that lead them to consciously eat fewer calories in the first place. The food may also provide them with an immediate reward, which holds more power during stress than the delayed reward they perceive from watching their weight. People who do not count calories or worry about their diet may refrain from overeating during stress simply because it will not work as a distraction for them.

A 2007 Kings College of London study wanted to see if stress would change the **Body Mass Index (BMI)** of a group of 71 women in their early 40s who were studying to become nurse practitioners. The researchers looked at the women's cortisol levels, dietary restraint, bingeing, mood, eating attitudes, and their sense of control over the effects of stress to see if these factors could predict changes in BMI. All of them started out with normal BMIs. They were measured again 12 weeks later, during exams. In that time 40 (56 percent) had gained weight, 19 (27 percent) lost weight, and 12 (17 percent) had stayed the same.

The women who had a greater sense of control over the effects of stress were less likely to have increased their BMI. The group whose BMIs had increased also experienced bingeing and higher cortisol levels and a decrease in sense of control, dietary restraint, and concern about their weight.

The women with BMIs that had gone down as a result of exam stress had increased their dietary restraint. In other words, they were significantly more vigilant about how much they were eating. The researchers thought this result may relate to the positive feeling of control that many anorexics get from dieting.

Another study, conducted in 2005, studied women who had lost weight over a period of six months under doctor supervision. Researchers talked to the women nine, 12, and 18 months after losing the weight to determine whether their mood and stress level affected their eating habits. It turned out that both depression and stress caused the women to consume more calories and to eat foods higher in fat. This may explain **yo-yo dieting**, when people cyclically lose weight, gain it back, lose it again, and so on.

SIGNS OF STRESS

Weight gain and weight loss aren't the only effects of stress, of course. Here are some other signs that you may be having a problem managing stress, according to the American Academy of Family Physicians:

- feeling depressed, edgy, guilty or tired;
- having headaches, stomachaches, or trouble sleeping;
- laughing or crying for no reason;
- blaming others when bad things happen to you;
- not enjoying things that used to be fun; and
- feeling resentful.

Q & A

Question: Are there any early warning signs of stress?

Answer: Tightness in your shoulders and neck or clenching your hands into fists are two early warning signs that you're experiencing stress, according to the American Academy of Family Physicians. Other physical symptoms of stress include tiredness, headaches, back pain, and an upset stomach.

MANAGING STRESS

No one can eliminate stress. But it's a good idea to figure out how to cope with stress, especially since those who are better able to cope with stress are less likely to turn to high-fat foods to make themselves feel better.

One of the first things you can do to manage stress is to think about what is causing the stress and decide what you have control over and what you do not. Then, for those things over which you do have control, consider making changes to reduce your stress. For example, if you are always racing the clock to get to school on time, you can try getting up earlier. Eliminating the morning stress might make you feel better overall, even if you hate early mornings.

You should also look for ways to use up some of the excess energy that stress creates. Exercise is one way. You can also try meditation or relaxation exercises. Talking to a friend or someone you trust can also reduce your stress. Even if you cannot control the problem, talking gives you a release. Spending time doing enjoyable things is another positive use of your energy and a distraction from the things that are making you feel anxious and tense.

FIGHTING BACK

Stress, as discussed, can affect the way you eat. But it works the other way too. Eating healthy, well-balanced meals on a regular basis is one way to fight against the effects of stress, says the American Academy of Family Physicians. They also recommend that you cut back on caffeine, get enough sleep, and exercise regularly.

See also: Eating Disorders, Causes of; Nutrition and Nutritional Deficiencies; Peer Pressure; Weight Control

FURTHER READING

Gould, Roger. *Shrink Yourself: Break Free from Emotional Eating Forever.* Indianapolis: Wiley, 2007.

Seaward, Brian. *Hot Stones and Funny Bones: Teens Helping Teens Cope with Stress and Anger.* Deerfield Beach, Fla.: HCI Teens, 2002.

■ TREATMENT

All of the remedies used to relieve or cure an eating disorder. After being diagnosed as having an eating disorder, people often deny that there is a problem. It's as if they've been guarding a precious secret and it's been discovered. Once an eating disorder is identified, treatment is needed as quickly as possible. Health-care professionals can't afford to wait until the person with the problem is willing to seek help.

WHO IS INVOLVED IN RECOVERY?

Because eating disorders are complex mental disorders with physical symptoms and side effects, the **recovery** process involves a variety of experts—including **psychotherapists**, physicians, nutritionists, and nurses. Each has a distinct role to play in the recovery process.

A psychotherapist is a person trained to help people deal with emotional problems. He or she helps them resolve the emotional issues that brought about the disorder and those that have developed or worsened as a result of it. People with eating disorders often experience other emotional illnesses that require treatment as well.

Physicians deal with the physical problems associated with an eating disorder. In fact, a physician may be the first to diagnose an eating disorder.

Nutritionists help people learn new eating habits. They provide their clients with personalized plans that enable them to gain, lose, or maintain weight in a healthy way. Nurses check symptoms, monitor progress, answer questions, and keep patients feeling as well as possible.

These experts often play a long-term role in their patients' lives, because even after they've recovered, there is a risk of a **relapse**—a return to old habits. By maintaining an ongoing relationship with their patients, health-care professionals try to prevent relapses or at least recognize the signs of one early enough to do something about it.

Family and friends, wittingly or unwittingly, play a role in the recovery process, too. Their involvement can have a big impact on recovery.

FORMS OF TREATMENT

Health-care professionals have a variety of treatments to choose from. They evaluate each in terms of the patient and his or her particular needs. Often a mix of approaches works best.

Hospitalization vs. outpatient care

A primary care physician takes into account several factors in determining whether a patient requires hospitalization. The physician considers the patient's height and weight and how quickly he or she has been losing weight. The physician may also check body temperature, heart rate, and blood pressure. He or she may order a urine analysis and blood work.

The doctor then determines if there are immediate nutritional needs that must be met in the hospital through intravenous feeding (providing nutrition directly into the veins) or other threats to the patient's health that require immediate attention. Patients resistant to treatment may be sent to the psychiatric unit of the hospital.

If the condition is serious but not immediately life threatening, the physician may recommend a residential treatment center. If the eating disorder is caught early and the patient has family support, the physician may call for outpatient care—treatment at a hospital without a hospital stay.

There are different types of outpatient care. **Intensive outpatient therapy** (IOP) is a treatment plan in which a group of patients receives help for several hours at a time three or more days a week. **Partial hospital programs** (PHPs) are an option for people who need more structure, intervention, and supervision. The treatment plan can be stepped up or down as the patient's needs change.

Fact Or Fiction?

If people suspect that I have an eating disorder, they'll take me from my friends and family and send me away somewhere for "rehab."

The Facts: The earlier an eating disorder or the tendency toward an eating disorder is diagnosed, the less intrusive the recovery plan needs to be. Many people with eating disorders participate in treatment plans that allow them to attend school or work during the recovery process.

Psychotherapy

Psychotherapy is a form of treatment that involves discussions between a patient and a therapist. It can be done with a single patient or a group. The more motivated and ready for treatment a patient is, the more likely the therapy will be successful. It also works best for those whose disorder has been caught in an early stage, before the most serious health-related problems have surfaced.

Group psychotherapy is a form of treatment that involves discussions among a group of patients with the help of a therapist. It usually occurs in conjunction with individual psychotherapy at an outpatient treatment center, a psychiatric hospital, or other inpatient setting. Through group psychotherapy, people with eating disorders learn that they are not alone in their struggles. Patients are both supported and confronted by other patients who are dealing with similar problems. Their interactions can be powerful therapy.

Group psychotherapy also presents a risk. By talking to peers (people in one's own age group), someone in the early stages of an eating disorder may learn about and later try new destructive behaviors. To avoid such problems, the group leader tries to ensure that group members are at about the same stage in their treatment.

Q & A

Question: What is behavior modification?

Answer: Behavior modification is based on reward and punishment. Your parents may use a form of behavior modification when they promise to let you use the family car if you improve your grades or take the car away if your grades go down. Most behavior modification treatments for eating disorders occur in an inpatient setting. They are usually part of a treatment regimen that involves other forms of therapy. Behavior modification focuses on stopping unhealthy, **compulsive** habits in the present, unlike other forms of therapy that look to the past to identify the causes of an eating disorder.

Cognitive behavioral therapy (CBT) also focuses on the present. CBT is an effort to alter the attitudes that prompt unhealthy eating behaviors as a way of changing the behaviors. For example, the belief that eating even a single gram of fat will result in obesity may cause someone to restrict all fat from his or her diet. By acknowledging and changing that attitude, he or she can begin to develop a healthier

approach to eating. Education and goal-setting are major components of CBT.

Family therapy

Family therapy is a form of treatment in which the therapist works
with not only the patient but also members of his or her family.
This approach is important for several reasons. Even the most well-
meaning, caring parents need guidance on how to deal with a child
who is recovering from an eating disorder. Through family therapy,
they can learn how to support their child's treatment plan.

Second, the family often plays a role in the development of an eating disorder. Family therapy can help uncover some of the events or
feelings that may have precipitated the problem.

Family therapy can also help young patients feel secure in their
family life. As a result, when the time comes, they will be able to
leave home for college or to lead an independent, adult life.

In addition to family therapy, some parents participate in couples
therapy. They meet privately with a therapist to talk freely about their
challenges and struggles without burdening their child with information he or she doesn't need (or often want) to know.

FAMILY LIFE

Being a part of a family can be wonderful, annoying, therapeutic,
and dangerous, often all at the same time. Creating and maintaining
a healthy family life is critical to recovery, because family issues are
often at the root of eating disorders. When family members take an
active part in the process, the chances for recovery improve.

Along with participating in therapy, family members can help the
patient in a variety of ways. Meals may be one of the most difficult
times of the day for the family. Yet eating together as often as possible can be helpful, as long as the family avoids emotional issues
at mealtimes. Lunch or dinner is not the time to talk about problems in school. It is also not the time to discuss portion control or
fat and calories. After all, anyone with an eating disorder needs to
overcome an obsession with those things. It helps to plan meals as a
family, perhaps shop for food and then prepare the meal together.

Families can also help a person with an eating disorder develop
new interests and set aside time to enjoy activities. When speaking

to someone with an eating disorder, it is best to avoid mentioning his or her physical appearance. Focus instead on overall health and energy level. "You look like you're full of energy today" is better than "You look better now that you've gained some weight." Most important, family members need to be patient. Recovery tends to be a long process.

MEDICATIONS

At one time, medical experts were skeptical about using **psychopharmacological drugs**—drugs prescribed to relieve the symptoms of mental illnesses—to help treat eating disorders. Today those drugs are an acceptable and often beneficial element in the recovery process. Patients now have many options, and a psychiatrist with expertise in treating eating disorders can help determine the medication or combination of medications that will work best for them.

Depression is often a component of eating disorders. Therefore a psychiatrist may recommend an **antidepressant**, which in turn may also relieve the need to **binge**, purge, or starve. Tricyclics are a class of antidepressants that have been used for decades. They increase the level of **neurotransmitters** (chemical "messengers") in the brain. Side effects include sedation, tiredness, dry mouth, constipation, **low blood pressure**, irregular heartbeats, and confusion.

Sometimes food cravings have a physiological root. The neurotransmitter **serotonin** can affect both mood and the feeling that one is hungry or full. Low levels of serotonin may be responsible for not only the urge to binge or purge but also depression. There are several drugs that help increase the serotonin level. They're called selective serotonin reuptake inhibitors (SSRIs). One SSRI, Prozac (fluoxetine), is often prescribed in low doses to help overcome depression and in higher doses to relieve the urge to binge. It is the only drug licensed specifically for treating bulimia.

Anxiety—fear or uneasiness about an anticipated event—is another common problem for people with eating disorders. Anxiety may be part of the reason for the disorder or it may be a result of efforts to develop healthier eating habits. Benzodiazepines are a class of antianxiety medication that helps people feel calmer. Side effects include drowsiness, confusion, inability to think clearly, and forgetfulness. These drugs become less effective over time, as the body develops a tolerance to them.

All of these drugs require ongoing medical supervision to ensure effectiveness and to deal with troublesome side effects.

SUPPORT GROUPS

Support groups bring together people with similar problems. They help participants feel less alone. Most support groups are free, and participants can usually join without giving their full names or details about who they are. There are also groups for friends and relatives of people with eating disorders.

Some support groups focus specifically on behaviors related to food. For example, participants may discuss not only the events that trigger their binges but also healthy alternatives to bingeing. Other groups deal with underlying emotional issues as well as specific behaviors associated with their disorder.

In addition to in-person support groups, telephone hotlines provide support and advice as needed, as do Internet chat rooms. In selecting a support network, it's important to choose ones that have well-documented experience. The National Association of Anorexia Nervosa and Associated Disorders is the oldest national nonprofit organization devoted to eating disorders. It is a good resource for finding support groups throughout the country.

Q & A

Question: My friend almost died from anorexia. Could a support group help her?

Answer: If she has a severe case of anorexia, your friend may have problems developing the relationships that make support groups effective. She also may still feel the desire to be thinner than everyone else, and therefore too competitive to provide and accept mutual support. The psychotherapist or physician helping your friend recover can let her know when a support group may be beneficial.

Teen support groups

Teenagers face unique challenges and social situations. A support group made up of teens may be beneficial in dealing with issues related to adolescence. Being among people of the same age can counterbalance peer pressure, especially when peer pressure has played a role in the development of an eating disorder. Teens speak the same language and they typically don't accept each other's excuses, which can be helpful in the recovery process. Local experts and national resource centers can refer people to teen support groups.

Overeaters Anonymous
Alcoholics Anonymous (AA) is one of the most successful self-help groups in the nation. **Overeaters Anonymous** (OA) models its philosophy after AA, taking the approach that binge eaters are as powerless over food as alcoholics are over liquor. Like AA, OA has a **12-step program** that requires participants to incorporate 12 specific rules into their lives to achieve lifelong recovery. Participants try to help one another resist the temptation to binge. Those who have been in the program for some time act as sponsors for people who are new to the program. Newcomers can call their sponsors to talk whenever they are finding it hard to resist the urge to binge. OA also has special meetings for people with bulimia and anorexia.

TEENS SPEAK

"Hello, My Name Is Jeannie and I Am a Bulimic."

Going to a support group was probably the hardest thing I've ever had to do. It was even harder than facing my parents and admitting I had been bulimic for two years. Luckily I didn't have too much time to think about it. My doctor told me about the group and said he'd scheduled me to attend a meeting the next day.

I didn't think I was going to be able to walk through the door. My whole body was shaking. My mom went with me to the group, but I had to go in by myself and face what I had become.

"Hello, my name is Jeannie and I am a bulimic. The last time I binged and purged was one week ago." Okay, so I really didn't have to say anything like that. I just went in, took a seat, and eased into the group.

In a way it was like the contrived situations you see on TV sitcoms or movies. The group welcomes the new person, saying, "Don't worry, we know where you're coming from." In another way, it was like being with friends late at night and getting to that point where everyone has something or someone to complain about. Only these weren't my friends; I didn't even know them.

Even though the atmosphere was casual, it was hard to open up at first. I would listen to someone talk and think, "I'm nothing like her." The more I listened, the more I realized that while my story was different from anyone else's, I also had things in common with these girls. I had the feeling they wouldn't judge me or condemn me for the things I'd done.

So I talked. I was wrong, actually. Some of them did sort of judge me—not in a bad way, though. What they did was hold me accountable. If they were going to make an effort to get over this, I had no excuse not to try as well.

SOCIAL LIFE

Recovery does not happen in a vacuum. It has to take place in all aspects of a person's life. Developing a comfortable social life is an important step in the recovery process.

DID YOU KNOW?

The Effectiveness of Treatment for Eating Disorders

Full recovery after treatment:	60%
Partial recovery after treatment:	20%
No improvement after treatment:	20%
Fatality rate after treatment:	2–3%
Fatality rate without treatment:	20%

Source: Anorexia Nervosa and Related Eating Disorders, Inc. (ANRED), 2007.

People with eating disorders rarely have much of a social life. Too often the eating disorder is used to avoid social situations, particularly if someone is troubled by a negative self-image. Or as an obsession with food and exercise mounts, the eating disorder can isolate a person from the social activities they once enjoyed.

Someone recovering from an eating disorder may find it helpful to ease their way into a social life by choosing activities that don't involve food. Eventually, however, establishing a healthy social life requires an ability and willingness to participate in all types of activities.

As this chart shows, treatment for an eating disorder often, but not always, leads to recovery. Treatment also significantly increases one's odds of surviving an eating disorder.

SCHOOL INVOLVEMENT

Schools can play an important role in helping to reduce eating disorders by providing students with opportunities to learn about eating disorders and understand their causes and symptoms. They can also help students deal with the media and other images that promote thinness and attractiveness by building their self-confidence.

For the student who is struggling with an eating disorder, the school environment may be safe or anxiety-ridden. Teachers and school administrators can help by being available to the student, providing information if the student wants it, and avoiding being confrontational.

RECOGNIZING AND CHANGING BEHAVIORS

Before people can change their behavior, they have to recognize that the behavior is causing a problem and then decide to solve that problem. These are the first steps to recovery. Then it becomes important to set small goals for oneself and recognize small improvements in behavior. For example, instead of thinking one has to stop vomiting completely, he or she might try to limit it to once a day, recognizing that doing so is a significant achievement. Once that's accomplished, the next goal can be little more ambitious.

Goal setting should not just involve food or purging. It should also include activities that will help develop a healthier lifestyle, perhaps joining a support group, having dinner with a friend, or attending a school activity. Goals should be simple and realistic, because achieving their goals gives people the strength to get better.

Some people find that keeping a journal of thoughts and feelings can be helpful during recovery. The journal can include writing, artwork, magazine clippings—anything that helps express feelings. A daily record is also a good idea. It may include eating disorder behaviors (bingeing, purging, taking medication, skipping a meal, etc.), food and beverage intake, and the emotions associated with each of these activities. Creating a daily or weekly meal plan can also be a good idea, because it can eliminate anxiety-producing decisions about food.

KEY ASPECTS OF TREATMENT

Successful treatment for eating disorders requires different types of experts and treatment methods to help overcome different aspects of the disorder. While treatment may be most successful with a willing patient, sometimes intervention is necessary before the patient is ready to admit to a problem.

See also: Anorexia; Bulimia; Eating Disorders, Causes of; Eating Disorders, Symptoms and Diagnosis of; Morbidity and Mortality; Peer Pressure; Self-Image

FURTHER READING

Apple, Robin F., and W. Stewart Agras. *Overcoming Your Eating Disorders: A Cognitive-Behavioral Therapy Approach for Bulimia Nervosa and Binge-Eating Disorder, Guided Self-Help Workbook.* New York: Oxford University Press, 2007.

Levenkron, Steven. *Anatomy of Anorexia.* New York: Lion's Crown, 2000.

Overeaters Anonymous. *The Twelve Steps and Ten Traditions of Overeaters Anonymous.* Rio Rancho, N.M.: Overeaters Anonymous, 1995.

Siegel, Michele, Ph.D, Judith Brisman, Ph.D, and Margot Weinshel, M.S.W. *Surviving an Eating Disorder: Strategies for Family and Friends.* New York: HarperCollins, 1997.

■ WEIGHT AND SOCIAL ACCEPTANCE

See: Ethnicity, Genetics, and Eating Disorders; Peer Pressure; Self-Image

■ WEIGHT CONTROL

Efforts to manage one's weight by developing healthy eating habits. Losing weight the healthy way—at a rate of one-half to two pounds a week—takes patience and will power. To lose 20 pounds may take at least two and a half months and perhaps as many as 10 months. Maintaining one's new weight after losing several pounds requires more than patience; it takes skill and a continued emphasis on healthy eating habits.

Some people want a quick or easy way to lose weight or avoid a weight gain. They want to eat whatever they want and then just erase the **calories**, like magic. Diet products and fad diets—many of them ineffective and some dangerous—are popular for that very reason. The problem with a quick weight loss is that whatever method is used, it's almost always unhealthy. Moreover, quick weight loss is usually followed by quick weight gain.

The best way to lose weight or avoid gaining weight is by changing one's eating habits. No food should be off-limits, but some foods (like candy and french fries) should be eaten rarely and in small portions. Otherwise, people should eat a **well-balanced diet** that includes a variety of foods. The more variety, the more likely one is to get all of the nutrients the body needs to grow, stay healthy, and protect itself against disease. The 2005 Dietary Guidelines—established by the U.S. Department of Agriculture and the Department of Health and Human Services—and MyPyramid.gov outline the components of a balanced diet and can help you figure out the foods you should include in your diet to be healthy.

Fact Or Fiction?

Weight loss is easy.

The Facts: Healthy weight loss is a slow process that takes patience and requires a change in eating habits. You have to pay attention to what you eat and make sure you are making healthy choices. You also have to make time for regular exercise. Anyone who says this kind of dieting is easy is lying. Even unhealthy weight loss isn't easy. Fad diets and diet products may spur quicker weight loss, but in the process you may experience such physical side effects as dizziness, fatigue, and stomach pain. To make matters worse, the weight will probably come back as soon as you stop the diet.

WHO IS OVERWEIGHT?

More than 17 percent of American children and teens (ages six to 19) are **overweight** and more than 32 percent of adults (over the age of 20) are **obese**—adding up to more than 84 million Americans in all. What about you? If you are among those Americans, ask your doctor about developing healthier eating habits. Serious weight problems shouldn't be ignored, because they can cause both physical and emotional problems.

If you believe you are overweight, but your doctor hasn't expressed concern, you should discuss the matter with him or her. Many people do not see themselves objectively. Attempting to lose weight if it is not necessary to do so is no healthier than carrying around extra weight.

If you can't talk to a doctor, use the **body mass index (BMI)** to see how much extra body fat you have. BMI-for-age charts and calculators can be found on the Centers for Disease and Prevention (CDC) Web site. To figure out where you fall on the BMI scale, once you are an adult, multiply your weight in pounds by 703. Divide that product by your height in inches and then divide that quotient by your height in inches again. (If you want to avoid the math, consult the BMI chart on page 139 of this book or use the BMI calculator on the Internet at www.nhlbisupport.com/bmi/bmicalc.htm.)

If your BMI falls between 18.5 and 25, you're in the normal range for your height and age. If your BMI is 25 to 30, you may be overweight and should talk to your doctor. A BMI of over 30 signals a dangerously high proportion of body fat—a serious medical problem. Obesity can lead to heart disease, **stroke, high blood pressure, diabetes,** gallbladder disease, gout (pain in your joints), sleep apnea, osteoarthritis, and cancer.

BMIs are not always accurate, especially if you are very muscular. In that case, the BMI is measuring excess muscle, not fat. It can also be inaccurate if you have experienced severe muscle loss. The index may then underestimate your body fat and incorrectly place you in a healthy range.

Q & A

Question: My doctor says I'm at a healthy weight, but I think I would look and feel better if I were thinner. Who is right?

Answer: If you look at the BMI scale, you'll notice that it provides range of weights for each height. For example, if you are 5'5", your weight would be considered healthy if it fell between 111 and 149 pounds. That's a large range. If you're at the higher end and want to exercise and modify your eating habits to reach a lower point within that range, that's okay. Just be sure to lose weight in a healthy way. Don't become compulsive about hitting a certain number on the scale.

CHRONIC WEIGHT LOSS

Experts say that chronic weight loss can be intentional or unintentional. Both have consequences.

Intentional weight loss

Those who experience chronic **intentional weight** loss are constantly on a diet. Their continuous efforts to lose weight may be a sign of an eating disorder. Anorexia and bulimia are common causes of chronic intentional weight loss. Anyone suffering from either disorder should seek medical attention as soon as possible.

Unintentional weight loss

Unintentional weight loss occurs when someone loses weight without trying. Such a loss is usually due to a problem in the endocrine or gastrointestinal system, a psychiatric disorder, nutritional deficiencies, an infection, a tumor, or a neurological disorder. The glands in the **endocrine system** release chemical messengers called **hormones** that regulate many bodily functions. **Hyperthyroidism** (when the thyroid produces too many hormones) is an example of a malfunction in the endocrine system that can cause weight loss.

The gastrointestinal system, which includes your stomach, intestines, gallbladder, and liver, regulates digestion, but chronic weight loss problems may start in the mouth. For example, someone may lose weight without trying because he or she has sores in the mouth or orthodontic braces that make it difficult or painful to eat. Chronic stomach pain might also result in a weight loss. Severe pulmonary problems, liver disease, kidney disease, and heart failure are also known to cause a drop in weight.

Depression is probably the most common psychiatric disorder that results in chronic unintentional weight loss. (It can also cause chronic weight gain. Depression affects different people in different ways.) People may also lose weight unintentionally if they smoke or abuse drugs. Former drug abusers suffering from withdrawal are also likely to experience weight loss. A number of medications, particularly thyroid medications, drugs used for chemotherapy, and overuse of laxatives, can also lead to weight loss.

Malnutrition is a health problem caused by the lack of the vitamins and minerals necessary to keep the body healthy or too many vitamins. Weight loss, as you might expect, is a common symptom of malnutrition. Anemia, a condition that occurs when there is not enough iron in the diet, can also cause weight loss. So can infections, such as tuberculosis or HIV, and cancer.

The treatment for chronic unintentional weight loss depends on the underlying cause. Options may include anything from **psychotherapy** to nutritional counseling to tube feeding.

DEVELOPING LIFELONG HABITS

Since unintentional weight loss can be a sign of a medical problem, it should not be treated lightly. Still, for anyone who has ever struggled to control his or her weight, it may sound like an enviable problem. Developing healthy eating and exercise habits at a young age is worth the time. Those habits could lead to less time spent on weight control later in life, and a longer life.

See also: Anorexia; Bulimia; Caloric Intake and Expenditures; Diet Pills; Nutrition and Nutritional Deficiencies; Obesity

■ WOMEN AND EATING DISORDERS

At least eight million people in the United States have an eating disorder, and 90 percent of them—approximately 7 million—are women, according to the National Association of Anorexia Nervosa and Associated Disorders (ANAD). The group also found that 86 percent of eating disorders occur by the age of 20. The National Eating Disorders Association (NEDA) estimates the incidence of eating disorders among women to be even higher, with 10 million women suffering from anorexia and bulimia and millions more suffering from binge-eating disorder.

Those numbers sound large and frightening. Keep in mind that overall, only a small minority of people develop eating disorders. Yet it's certainly significant that so many of the people who do get eating disorders are female.

According to health-care professionals who treat eating disorders, more and more older patients, women in their 40s and 50s, are experiencing relapses or are being diagnosed with an eating disorder for the first time.

To understand why, walk through a shopping mall. You'll see a huge selection of stylish clothing and accessories for young girls. There is an even larger selection for older women as well as an overabundance of makeup, skin-care products, hair-coloring products, and more.

The message is clear. It is a message that Hollywood reinforces. Many celebrities in their 40s, 50s, and even 60s seem ageless. Although most of them spend huge amounts of money and time to maintain their youthful appearance, they inspire other women to want to be just as thin and as beautiful.

The result is that many females focus on their physical appearance from an early age and continue to do so throughout their lives. Some come to believe that physical beauty matters deeply and that being thin is a sign of beauty. Although such attitudes can contribute to many eating disorders, they are not the only reason many women develop eating disorders. Some do so as a part of an effort to take control of their lives. For others, it is a response to a major transition in their life or an attempt to live up to someone else's expectations.

RATES

Approximately 0.5 percent to 1 percent of young women will suffer anorexia, according to Sarah Pritts and Jeffrey Susman, coauthors of a 2003 article on eating disorders in *American Family Physician*. Many more will develop bulimia. Several studies done in the 1990s estimated that bulimia affects 2 to 5 percent of young women. A large national 2007 survey on adults published in *Biological Psychiatry* found that 0.9 percent of women reported having had anorexia, and 1.5 percent of women reported having had bulimia sometime in their lives.

The next area for research may center specifically on the prevalence of eating disorders among middle-aged women. There are no national studies on the subject as yet. However, eating disorder specialists at two of the largest treatment centers in the United States have offered anecdotal evidence that eating disorders are rising among women in their 40s, 50s, and 60s.

The reasons for the rise are not yet known, but it could be the result of a combination of factors including **anxiety** about aging, hormonal changes, demographics (there has been a rise in the number of middle-aged women in the current population), and an increased awareness of the importance of seeking treatment.

CAUSES

There are many different causes of eating disorders among women, including low **self-esteem**, depression, loneliness, **perfectionist** tendencies, family issues, and a history of sexual, physical, or emotional abuse. Researchers believe genetics can also increase vulnerability to an eating disorder. The emphasis in American society on physical beauty, thinness, dieting, and exercise plays a role in the prevalence of eating disorders as well.

In young adolescent girls, eating disorders are often triggered by conflicting feelings about growing up and going through puberty. Girls may be frightened of getting older, having increased independence, and attracting boys and men who may place sexual demands on them. Anorexia can slow or even stop sexual development. Instead of developing womanly curves that include breasts and hips, the body of a teenager with anorexia remains childlike.

Women's bodies also change during middle age. **Metabolism** slows, **hormone** levels change, and menopause approaches. Each may trigger an eating disorder. As women age, they may become less independent. Older women who feel frustrated by the need to rely on the care of others may develop eating disorders in an attempt to regain some element of control over their lives.

FEMALES COMPARED TO MALES

While there is societal pressure for males to be strong, muscular, and fit, the pressure for women is to be thin. In 1992, a study published in the *International Journal of Eating Disorders* reported that women's magazines had more than 10 times as many ads and articles promoting weight loss as men's magazines. A 12-year study published by the same journal in 1994 found many more body-oriented articles in women's magazines than those for men. Similar studies have focused on television and movies, all with the same basic findings. One study, published in the *Psychology of Women Quarterly* in 2007, focused on whether social pressure to conform would lead to an increased incidence of eating disorders among college women living in sorority houses. The researchers surveyed 265 college women and found that sororities tended to attract women who were at risk of developing an eating disorder and that living in a sorority house did increase the likelihood of having an eating disorder. Both in the media and among their peers, American girls and women are continuously confronted with images of thin women, and few feel that they can measure up to those images.

An important difference between males and females with eating disorders is the rate at which they seek treatment. With increased awareness of how deadly eating disorders can be, the overall number of people who get treatment has increased, but women seek treatment much more often than men.

Social expectations may explain why women are more likely to seek treatment. For many years, eating disorders were considered a female problem. Even though experts now know that men suffer from eating disorders, it is still more socially acceptable for a woman to admit to a debilitating disorder centered on issues related to food and weight.

There have also been very few treatment programs designed specifically for men, although that is slowly changing. Rogers Memorial Hospital in Wisconsin runs an eating disorders treatment program specifically for boys and men, which includes an all-male residential center and male-only therapy groups.

Q & A

Question: I heard some girls talking about logging on to "pro ana" and "pro mia" Web sites. What are they?

Answer: You can go to the Internet and find many Web sites that help people understand the dangers of eating disorders and offer support in the recovery process. Unfortunately, some people have also set up what are known as "pro ana" and "pro mia" Web sites—Web sites that consider anorexia and bulimia a lifestyle rather than an illness. These Web sites are dangerous, and anyone spending time on them needs the help of an eating disorders specialist.

PREVENTION

The National Eating Disorders Association was created in 2001, when Eating Disorders Awareness and Prevention (EDAP) and the American Anorexia Bulimia Association (AABA) formed what they call "the largest eating disorders prevention and advocacy organization in the world." Their activities include a national program called GO GIRLS! (Giving Our Girls Inspiration and Resources for Lasting Self-Esteem). It brings together adolescent girls for group discussions that strengthen their self-image. The girls also try to encourage the media and retailers to promote positive body images. The main goal of the group is to prevent eating disorders.

CALLING IT A "WOMAN'S PROBLEM"

The fact that eating disorders may be more accepted among girls and women is both bad and good. On the negative side, eating disorders among females carry less of a stigma because so many women are affected. On the positive side, that acceptance may encourage more women to seek treatment, and early treatment is crucial to survival.

See also: Anorexia; Bulimia; Eating Disorders, Causes of; Eating Disorders in Men and Boys; Media and Eating Disorders; Morbidity and Mortality; Stress and Eating Habits

FURTHER READING
Yancey, Diane. *Eating Disorders.* Brookfield, Conn.: Twenty-First Century Books, 1999.

HOTLINES
AND HELP SITES

The Alliance for Eating Disorders Awareness
URL: http://www.eatingdisorderinfo.org
Phone: 1-866-662-1235
Affiliation: Eating Disorders Coalition for Research, Policy and Action
  (EDC), a cooperative of professional and advocacy-based organizations committed to advancing the federal recognition of eating
  disorders as a public health priority
Mission: to allow children and young adults the opportunity to learn
  about eating disorders and the positive effects of a healthy body
  image; eating-disorders awareness programs on a nationwide
  basis; also provides educational information about the warning
  signs, dangers, and consequences of anorexia, bulimia, and other
  related disorders

American Dietetic Association (ADA)
URL: http://www.eatright.org
Phone: 1-800-877-1600
Mission: provides a wealth of nutrition information, including locat-
  ing nutritionists by zip code

Anorexia Nervosa and Related Eating Disorders, Inc. (ANRED)
URL: http://www.anred.com
Affiliation: National Eating Disorders Association; run by health pro-
  fessionals actively involved in the field of eating disorders
Mission: to provide information food and weight disorders
Program: information about anorexia nervosa, bulimia nervosa,
  binge-eating disorder, and other food and weight disorders; material

includes self-help tips and information about recovery and prevention; Web site is updated monthly

Center for Change
URL: http://www.centerforchange.com
Phone: 1-888-224-8250
Mission: to provide care for people with eating disorders in an atmosphere of care and trust
Program: information about a variety of eating disorders, treatment options, and the treatment plans available at the center

Eating-Disorder.com
URL: http://www.eating-disorder.com
Phone: 1-866-575-8179
Mission: to provide users with information on finding eating disorder treatment centers and mental health professionals

GO GIRLS! (Giving Our Girls Inspiration and Resources for Lasting Self-Esteem)
URL: http://www.nationaleatingdisorders.org/p.asp?WebPage_ID=296
Phone: 1-206-382-3587
Affiliation: National Eating Disorders Association
Mission: to promote responsible advertising and to advocate for positive body images of youth by the media and major retailers
Program: high school prevention program and curriculum that involves high school girls working together to improve self-esteem and body image while acting as a voice for change

MEDLINEplus Health Information
URL: http://www.nlm.nih.gov/medlineplus
Affiliation: U.S. National Library of Medicine and the National Institutes of Health
Mission: to provide information on more than 600 health topics
Program: includes information on drugs, a medical encyclopedia and dictionary, current health news, directory of experts and resources, and more

National Association of Anorexia Nervosa and Associated Disorders (ANAD)
URL: http://www.anad.org
Phone: 1-847-831-3438 (9:00 A.M. to 5:00 P.M. Central Time, M–F)

Mission: dedicated to alleviating the problems of eating disorders and promoting healthy lifestyles

Program: provides hotline counseling, a national network of free support groups, referrals to health professionals, and education and prevention programs

National Eating Disorders Association (NEDA)
URL: http://www.nationaleatingdisorders.org
Phone: 1-800-931-2237

Affiliation: formed when Eating Disorders Awareness & Prevention joined forces with the American Anorexia Bulimia Association; also formed alliances with Anorexia Nervosa and Related Disorders, Inc., and the National Eating Disorders Organization

Mission: dedicated to expanding public understanding of eating disorders and promoting access to quality treatment for those affected as well as support for their families

Program: education, advocacy, and research

National Institutes of Health
URL: http://www.nimh.nih.gov/health/topics/eatingdisorders/index.shtml

Mission: conduct research programs on health issues across the board, maintain informational resources, enhance the country's well-being through science; keep the public informed on pressing health issues, such as eating disorders

Nutrition and Your Health: Dietary Guidelines for Americans
URL: http://www.health.gov/dietaryguidelines
Phone: 1-888-878-3256

Affiliation: Department of Health and Human Services and the Department of Agriculture

Mission: to provide authoritative advice for people two years and older about how good dietary habits can promote health and reduce risk for major chronic diseases, and to serve as the basis for federal food and nutrition education programs; includes a BMI chart and MyPyramid; dietary guidelines updated every five years

Overeaters Anonymous
URL: http://www.overeatersanonymous.org
Phone: 1-505-891-2664
Mission: to help its members stop compulsive overeating

186 The Truth About Eating Disorders

Programs: meetings and other tools that provide a fellowship of experience, strength, and hope; members support one another's anonymity

Rader Programs
URL: http://www.raderprograms.com
Phone: 1-800-841-1515
Mission: help individuals help themselves recover from the effects of an eating disorder
Programs: provides acute and day-care treatment for people suffering from eating disorders; centers in California and Oklahoma

The Renfrew Center
URL: http://www.renfrewcenter.com
Phone: 1-800-RENFREW
Affiliation: the Renfrew Foundation residential facility
Mission: dedicated exclusively to the treatment of eating disorders
Program: center provides information and treatment for women with eating disorders; foundation develops and implements programs that advance the awareness of eating disorders and related issues, and provides financial assistance for women who cannot afford professional treatment

Something Fishy
URL: http://www.something-fishy.org
Phone: 1-866-690-7239
Mission: dedicated to increasing awareness of eating disorders and encouraging recovery
Program: provides information, treatment options and referrals, online support, and chats

WebMD
URL: http://my.webmd.com
Affiliation: WebMD maintains objective editorial control but is funded by a variety of associations and corporate sponsors
Mission: to provide a comprehensive online resource for health information
Program: includes interactive calculators and quizzes, a medical library, drug information, slide shows, symptom matching, and more

Youth Risk Behavior Surveillance System
URL: http://www.cdc.gov/nccdphp/dash/yrbs
Affiliation: Centers for Disease Control's National Center for Chronic Disease Prevention and Health Promotion
Mission: to monitor priority health risk behaviors that contribute markedly to the leading causes of death, disability, and social problems among youth and adults in the United States
Program: conducts surveys of ninth- through 12th-grade students every two years

GLOSSARY

acculturation   the process of adapting to a new culture or blending cultures

addiction, addictions   psychological, emotional, or physical dependence on something

aerobic exercise or exercises   vigorous, repetitive exercise, such as walking, running, or swimming, that increases breathing, raises the heart rate, and uses up oxygen in your blood

allergen, allergens   a substance that triggers the immune system to respond inappropriately or harmfully

anabolic steroids   synthetic substances related to male sex hormones, prescribed to treat specific medical conditions but often abused, illegally, by athletes seeking to build muscle and improve their performance

anaphylaxis   a severe and sometimes deadly allergic reaction

anemia   a deficiency in red blood cells, hemoglobin, or total volume

antibodies   proteins produced by the body's **immune system** as part of its defense against foreign bacteria or blood cells

antidepressant, antidepressants   medications used to treat depression

antioxidants   chemicals from plants, including vitamin C and vitamin E, which protect cells and tissues from being damaged by oxidation

anxiety   feelings of worry, fear, and unease

basal metabolic rate   measurement of energy used when the body is at rest

behavioral therapy   therapy that focuses on changing current behaviors instead of exploring underlying emotional issues

binge   to consume huge amounts of food in a short amount of time

bipolar disorder   a psychological condition in which the patient's moods swing between "mania," when he or she feels full of energy and (usually) confidence, and deep depression or sadness

body composition   percentage of body fat and lean body mass (bones, muscles, and organs)

body dysmorphic disorder   a preoccupation with an imagined defect in physical appearance that causes distress and difficulty functioning in everyday social situations

body mass index (BMI)   a scale that uses a person's height and weight to assess body fat in order to determine whether he or she is at a healthy weight or is overweight or obese

bomb calorimeter   an instrument used to measure calories of food

calorie, calories   a measurement unit for energy

carbohydrates   one of the three main food groups (along with protein and fat) that gives the body energy; made up of sugars and starches that the body converts to glucose

cholesterol   a fat-like substance made by the body and found naturally in animal foods such as meat, fish, poultry, eggs, and dairy products; high levels of cholesterol can lead to heart disease

cognitive behavioral therapy   a treatment in which the therapist helps the patient find new ways of responding to "triggers" (for example, things that may prompt someone with bulimia or a binge-eating disorder to eat)

comorbidity   the simultaneous appearance of two or more illnesses in one person

complex carbohydrates   starches, such as bread, pasta, and beans, that the body breaks down into glucose

compulsive   feeling compelled to do something over and over

compulsive exercise, compulsive exerciser   a form of purging calories in which someone exercises way too much, to the point that it is mentally and physically unhealthy; also called anorexia athletica and obligatory exercise

cortisol   a hormone produced by the body when under stress

dehydration   lack of fluids in the body

delusions   false beliefs held despite evidence to the contrary

diabetes   a disease in which the body cannot use blood glucose as energy because it has too little **insulin** or does not process insulin properly

dietary supplements   products developed from natural sources that are intended or marketed to improve one's health in some way; also called herbal supplements or nutritional supplements

diuretics   chemicals that are intended to increase urination and get rid of excess fluid; some people with eating disorders abuse diuretics in an attempt to lose weight

dysthymia   a chronic form of depression in which the symptoms are less severe than in major depression and are ongoing rather than cyclical

electrocardiogram   a test, also called an EKG or ECG, that measures how the heart is functioning

electrolytes   sodium, potassium, and other minerals in the blood which help regulate the body's fluids

endocrine system   a system of ductless glands that regulate bodily functions through hormones secreted into the bloodstream

euphoria   a feeling of happiness, confidence, or well-being

family therapy   psychotherapy in which the patient and his or her spouse, parents, and/or children meet on a regular basis in order to help understand the problems associated with the cause and treatment of an eating disorder and to learn to get along better with one another

fat, fats   one of the three main food groups (along with carbohydrates and protein) that give the body energy; fats are the most concentrated source of energy in foods

food-induced allergy   a negative response by the immune system to a food that is harmless in most people

hallucination, hallucinations   a false sight or sound

healthy weight, healthy weight range   a **body mass index** that falls between 18.5 and 25

high blood pressure   when the pressure of the blood on the blood vessels is higher than normal, which increases risk of heart disease and stroke; also called hypertension

histamines   substances released by the cells in the body after coming in contact with allergens; cause of allergic symptoms such as rashes, runny noses, and wheezing

homeostasis   the body's process of maintaining equilibrium; for example, eating because one's energy level is low

hormone, hormones   a chemical that some cells in the body release to help other cells work; for example, insulin is a hormone that helps the body use glucose as energy

hyperthyroidism   when the thyroid releases too many of its hormones

hypothalamus   part of the brain that controls hunger, thirst, and body temperature

immune system   the cells and organs in the body that fight disease and infection

insulin   the hormone that regulates the level of glucose (sugar) in the body

intensive outpatient therapy   a form of treatment for eating disorders in which the patient lives at home and goes to a hospital, clinic, or treatment center for treatment several hours at a time several days a week; also called IOP

intentional weight loss   a situation in which one purposely eats fewer calories and/or increases their activity level in order to lose weight

Ipecac syrup   substance that is intended to be used to induce vomiting after accidentally ingesting a poisonous substance; some people with eating disorders use it to induce vomiting in an attempt to lose weight

ketones   chemical substances the body makes when it does not have enough insulin, which can occur if one fasts or goes on an unhealthy diet

ketosis   a buildup of ketones in the body, which can make a person very sick and is especially risky for pregnant women or people with diabetes; can be caused by a lack of carbohydrates

leptin   a hormone that is produced by fat cells and affects how the body regulates feelings of fullness and weight

lethargy   tiredness or lack of energy

lifestyle disease   a health condition associated with the way someone lives

lipase inhibitors   a new class of obesity drugs that reduce the amount of fat the body absorbs; approved by the Food and Drug Administration in 1999

low blood pressure   when the pressure of the blood on the blood vessels is lower than normal, causing one to feel dizzy and light-headed

major depression   the most severe form of depression, in which one exhibits a number of symptoms of depression at once and has difficulty meeting responsibilities and taking part in and enjoying everyday activities

malnutrition   a physical condition in which one's body does not have enough vitamins and minerals to stay healthy

metabolism   the physical and chemical processes in the body related to how the body generates and uses energy, including nutrition, digestion, absorption, elimination, respiration, circulation, and temperature regulation

neurochemistry   the study of chemicals in the body and how they affect the nervous system

neuroepinephrine   a neurotransmitter that gives one a sense of emotional and physical fulfillment

neurotransmitter, neurotransmitters   a chemical messenger that delivers information to the brain

nutritional rehabilitation   a form of treatment for bulimia that focuses on establishing a regular eating pattern

obese   having too much body fat; in adults, obesity is defined by a body mass index (BMI) above 30

obsessive-compulsive disorder   a form of anxiety characterized by recurring and intrusive thoughts, feelings, or ideas (obsessions) and/or the need to repeat certain patterns of behavior (compulsions)

omega-3 fatty acids   a type of polyunsaturated fat that has been shown to be beneficial to the heart; found in oily fish (such as tuna and salmon), dark green leafy vegetables, flaxseed, and some vegetable oils

organ failure a condition in which one of the major organs in the body, such as the heart or kidney, becomes unable to function

Overeaters Anonymous a self-help group for binge eaters and other overeaters that models itself after Alcoholics Anonymous and has a 12-step program to help members overcome their addiction to food

over-the-counter (OTC) refers to drugs that can be purchased at a store without a prescription

overweight a condition in which one is outside the healthy weight range and has a **body mass index** of 25 to 30

paranoid distrusting others out of an irrational sense that people are out to harm oneself

partial hospital programs a form of treatment for eating disorders in which the patient lives at home but attends all-day treatment at a hospital or treatment center; also called PHP

perfectionist feeling compelled to set and attempt to attain extremely high standards; a common personality type among people with eating disorders

post-traumatic stress disorder mental illness characterized by anxiety that develops after an extremely troublesome or frightening ordeal

protein, proteins one of the three main food groups (along with carbohydrates and fats) that gives the body energy; animal products provide complete sources of protein, and some grains, fruits, and vegetables provide incomplete proteins

psychiatrist, psychiatrists a medical doctor who specializes in mental, emotional, or behavioral disorders

psychopharmacological drugs drugs that affect the brain and central nervous system and relieve the symptoms of mental illnesses; also called psychotropic medications

psychosis a psychological condition characterized by hallucinations, delusions, or other major mental dysfunction

psychosocial intervention a form of treatment for bulimia that involves individual and/or group psychotherapy in an effort to determine underlying emotional problems, improve self-esteem, and change attitudes about food, weight, and appearance

psychotherapist, psychotherapists a therapist who helps people overcome mental and emotional disorders

psychotherapy a course of treatment, often based on discussion between a patient and a doctor or counselor, aimed at helping the patient modify their behavior and/or improve their mental state

recovery the process of becoming free of the symptoms of a disease

relapse, relapses a reoccurrence of the symptoms of an eating disorder, following a period of improvement

remission a reduction or disappearance of the signs and symptoms of a disease or disorder

risk factor or factors anything, such as family background or personal problems, that raises the chances of a person developing a disease or disorder

Rubenesque a term used to describe large women, which was derived from the artwork of Peter Paul Rubens; Rubens was a master painter famous for his 17th-century portraits of full-figured nude women.

saturated fat or fats fats that are found in animal products (butter, cheese, whole milk, ice cream, cream, and fatty meats), as well as in coconut, palm, and palm kernel oils; these fats raise the level of "bad cholesterol" in the blood and should be consumed as rarely as possible

self-esteem the sense of value one attributes to oneself

serotonin a neurotransmitter that affects a person's mood and feelings of being hungry or full

shock weakened body function that can be caused by blood loss, trauma, severe infection, an allergic reaction, or, in diabetics, a drop in blood sugar

simple carbohydrates sugars that the body breaks down into glucose

stroke an interruption of the blood supply to any part of the brain, causing brain damage

suicide, suicides killing oneself

supplements pills, powders, or liquids containing vitamins, minerals, or proteins that are meant to affect one's health in some way

support group or groups a group of people with a common problem who help one another by sharing information and personal experiences

therapeutic related to the treatment or cure of disease

trans fats unhealthy form of fat used in many processed foods; also known as partially hydrogenated fats

12-step program any treatment program for alcoholism, overeating, or other addictions that stresses the 12 steps to recovery developed by Alcoholics Anonymous

underweight having a BMI less than 18.5

unintentional weight loss a condition in which one loses weight without trying; typically indicates the presence of some physical or mental health problem

unsaturated fats fats that help to lower blood cholesterol if used in place of saturated fats; even unsaturated fats should be consumed in limited quantities because of their high calorie count; monounsaturated and polyunsaturated fats are both types of unsaturated fats

vegans   vegetarians who do not consume any dairy products

well-balanced diet   a diet that includes a wide variety of foods and only a very limited amount of sweets and saturated fats

yo-yo dieting   trying different diets or the same diet over and over in an effort to lose weight rather than sticking to one consistent eating plan

INDEX

Page numbers in *italic* indicate graphs or sidebars. Page numbers in **bold** denote main entries.

A

AA 170
AABA 181
AAFP 60, 98, 123, 160, 162–163
acculturation 78–79
ADA. *See* American Dietetic Association (ADA)
ADHD 54, 124
Adipex-P 51
adoption studies 80
advertising 94–95, 116–117
aerobics 89
African Americans 76–78, 143
alcohol abuse 69
Alcoholics Anonymous (AA) 170
allergies, food. *See* food allergies
Allī 51
Alliance for Eating Disorders Awareness 183
American Academy of Family Physicians (AAFP) 60, 98, 123, 160, 162–163
American Anorexia Bulimia Association (AABA) 181
American Cancer Society 137–138
American Diabetes Association 92
American Dietetic Association (ADA)
  contact information 183
  on depression 48

on dietary guidelines 40
on fad diets 91, 92, 93, 95
on obesity 140–141
American Heart Association 92
American Journal of Human Genetics 81
American Journal of Psychiatry
  on bulimia 33
  on males and eating disorders 72
  on morbidity and mortality rates 122, 124
  on purging 150
American Psychiatric Association
  on anxiety disorders and eating disorders 54
  on binge-eating disorder 30
  on bulimia 32
  on morbidity and mortality rates 122
American Psychological Association (APA) 153
ANAD. *See* National Association of Anorexia Nervosa and Associated Disorders (ANAD)
Andersen, R.E. 73
anorexia 15–21
  behavioral patterns of 64
  defined 2
  genetics and 81

health problems associated with
17
helping a friend with 19
mortality rates of 122
obesity and 82–83
reasons for 16
signs of 4, 16–17, 63
statistics of 15
treatment of 18–19
weight loss, absence of 18
Anorexia Nervosa and Related
Eating Disorders, Inc. (ANRED) 10,
54
  bigorexia 24
  binge-eating disorder 28
  contact information 183–184
  family life 69
  morbidity and mortality rates 123
ANRED. *See* Anorexia Nervosa
and Related Eating Disorders, Inc.
(ANRED)
antidepressants 18–19, 36, 48, 168
anxiety disorders 54, 168
APA 153
Archives of General Psychiatry 32,
81, 107
Asian Americans 77–78
athletics 73, 88, 123
Atkins Diet 92
attention-deficit/hyperactivity
disorder (ADHD) 54, 124

B

Becker, Anne 47, 58
behavioral patterns 1–12
  changes in 5
  defined 2
  secrecy 4, 5, 29
  as signs of eating disorders 64–65
behavioral therapy 18
behavior modification 166–167,
172–173. *See also* treatment
Berners-Lee, Tim 103
bigorexia 21–25
  body image and 25

dangers of 23
drug use and 24–25
identifying 22
mentioned 6
binge-eating disorder **25–31**
  behavioral patterns of 65
  depression and 31
  mentioned 2
  mortality rates and 122–123
  signs of 5, 28–29, 64
  statistics of 28
  treatment of 29–30
bingeing. *See* binge-eating disorder;
bulimia
Biological Psychiatry
  on anorexia 15
  on binge-eating disorder 28
  on bulimia 150
  on males and eating disorders 71
  on morbidity and mortality rates
  121–122, 123
  on women and eating disorders,
  statistics on 178
bipolar disorder 43
BMI. *See* body mass index (BMI)
body dysmorphic disorder 22. *See
also* bigorexia
body fat 139–140. *See also* body
mass index (BMI)
body image 5–6, 25, 154–155. *See
also* self-image
body mass index (BMI) *139*
  assessing weight with 175
  average American woman and 58
  exercise and 90
  genetics and 80–81
  healthy weight range and 34
  obesity and 135–136, *138*
  and stress, effects of 161
body sculpting 89
*Body Wars: Making Peace with
Women's Bodies* (Maine) 93
Bontril 51
Brownell, Kelly 117
Bulik, Cynthia M. 54, 56, 81

bulimia 31–38
  behavioral patterns of 65
  defined 2
  genetics and 81
  mortality rates and 122–123
  signs of 4–5, 33–34, 63–64
  statistics of 32–33
  treatment of 36

C

Caldwell, Paul 69
caloric intake and expenditures 38–42. *See also* exercise; fad diets; nutrition and nutritional deficiencies; weight control
Canadian Journal of Psychology 23
cancer 137–138
CBT 19, 166–167
CDC. *See* Centers for Disease Control and Prevention (CDC)
Center for Change 184
Centers for Disease Control and Prevention (CDC)
  exercise 86
  mentioned 3, 119
  nutrition and nutritional deficiencies 125, 126–127
  on obesity 136, 137
Chao, Y. May 71
Chavanu, Bakari 116
Clinical Psychology Review 19
cognitive behavioral therapy (CBT) 19, 166–167
Counseling Center for Human Development 155–156
Cuban Americans 79

D

depression 42–49. *See also* antidepressants; suicide
  binge-eating disorder and 31
  effects of 49
  genetic nature of 45–46
  high school students and *44*
  symptoms of 44–45

and weight loss/gain 46, 47, 176–177
Desoxyn 51
DHHS (U.S. Department of Health and Human Services) 83, 125–126, 139, 174
diabetes 60, 64, 85
Dietary Guidelines for Americans (USDA) 83. *See also* MyPyramid
dieting. *See* caloric intake and expenditures; diet pills; fad diets
diet pills 49–53, 50–51, 51–53. *See also* medications
drug abuse 24–25. *See also* laxative abuse
dysthymia 43

E

Eating-Disorder.com 184
eating disorders 69–70, 147. *See also specific disorders and topics*
  diagnosis of 7–8
  effects of 8–10
  health problems associated with 9–10
  helping a friend with 19, 70, 147
  history of 61
  signs/symptoms of 3–5
  statistics of 10
  testing for 67–69
  trends, recent 147–148
  Westernization of 148
Eating Disorders (journal) 77, 78
eating disorders, causes of 54–62
  family influences 55–56
  genetics 56–57
  individual traits 60
  media expectations 58–59
  physical conditions 59–60
  psychological difficulties 54–55
  social influences 57–58
  social skills 55
eating disorders, symptoms and diagnosis of 62–71. *See also* eating disorders, causes of
  behavioral patterns 64–65

emotional responses 69
family traits 69
physical signs 62–63
psychological assessment 68–69
self-perception 69–70
social patterns 66
Eating Disorders Awareness and
 Prevention (EDAP) 181
Eating Disorders Coalition 121
eating disorders in men and boys
 71–75. *See also* women and eating
 disorders
  bigorexia and 22
  bulimia and 32–33, 150
  causes of 73
  eating disorders and 3, 15
  females, males compared 179–
   180
  research on 75
  statistics of 71–72
  treatment options for 180
Eating Disorders Review 56
eating patterns
  depression and 48
  of high school students 128
  stress and 158–163
EDAP 181
emotional eating 160–162
Essence (magazine) 77
Etcoff, Nancy 117
ethnicity and eating disorders
 75–83
European Eating Disorders Review
 10
exercise **83–90.** *See also* caloric
 intake and expenditures; obesity;
 weight control
  abnormal practices 87–88
  addiction to 88
  benefits of 84, 90
  calories burned during 41, 85
  evaluating time spent 23
  health problems and 9
  healthy practices 83–85
high school student participation
 in 85
overview 6–7
weight and physical activity 89–
 90

F

fact or fiction
  addiction and eating disorders 60
  alcohol 49
  anorexia 16, 17–18
  bulimia 34
  caloric intake 39
  depression 43–44, 49
  diet pills 53
  eating disorders, symptoms and
   diagnosis of 68
  exercise 86, 88
  fad diets 91
  food allergies 102
  Internet 105
  laxatives, herbal 110–111
  males and eating disorders 72–73
  media and eating disorders 114,
   115–116
  nutrition and nutritional
   deficiencies 128
  obesity 82, 136–137
  peer pressure 146
  steroids 24–25
  treatment 165
  weight control 174
fad diets **90–98.** *See also* caloric
 intake and expenditures; diet pills;
 weight control
  Atkins Diet 92
  fasting 93–94
  high-fiber, low-calorie diets 93
  high-protein, low-carbohydrate
   diets 92
  magic-food diets 91–92
  meal-replacement diets 93
  media and 94–96
  obesity and 140

South Beach Diet 92
  types of 91–94
family life 55–56, 167–168
family therapy 167
FANSA 96
fashion models. *See* models
fasting 93–94
fats, saturated and unsaturated
  127–128
FDA 50–53, 99, 111
Federal Trade Commission (FTC)
  94–95
Fiji Island study 58–59
food allergies **98–103**
  about 98–100
  identifying 100–101
  treating 101–102
Food and Drug Administration (FDA)
  50–53, 99, 111
Food and Nutrition Science Alliance
  (FANSA) 96
Food Guide Pyramid 130–132, 174
Friedman, Jeffrey 82
FTC 94–95

G

gender issues. *See* eating disorders in
  men and boys; women and eating
  disorders
genetics **75–83**
  depression and 45–46
  eating disorders and 56–57
  obesity and 140–141
GO GIRLS (Giving Our Girls
  Inspiration and Resources for
  Lasting Self-Esteem) 147, 181, 184
guar gum 52

H

Harris Interactive poll 95
Harvard Eating Disorders Clinic 150
Health (magazine) 114
health problems
  anorexia and 17

binge-eating disorder and 29
  bulimia and 35–36
  and eating habits, poor 126–127
  fad diets and 91–94
  laxative abuse and 110
  obesity and 137–139, 175
  purging and 149–150
Healthy People 2010 36
Hirsch, Jules 81–83, 140
*Hispanic Journal of Behavioral
  Sciences* 79
Hispanics 78
homosexuals 72–73
hormones 57
hospitalization of eating disorder
  patients 165
hotlines and help sites 183–187
Hudson, James I. 28

I

IFIC 39, 95, 99, 129
International Food Information
  Council Foundation (IFIC) 39, 95,
  99, 129
*International Journal of Eating
  Disorders*
  on anorexia 19
  on ethnicity and eating disorders
    79
  on males and eating disorders 71
  on media and eating disorders 112
  on suicide and anorexia 122
  on women and eating disorders 179
International Journal of Men's Health
  23
Internet **103–108.** *See also* media
  and eating disorders
  benefits 105–107
  dangers 103–105
  as information source 95, 102
  media and 118–119
  teen usage 103
Ionamin 51
ipecac syrup 149

J

Journal of Adolescent Health 78
*Journal of Allergy and Clincal
Immunology* 102
Journal of Pediatrics 102
Journal of Research on Adolescence
114

K

Kaiser Family Foundation 103, 115,
118
Kaye, Walter H. 54, 81
Kelly, Christina 117–118
Kirkpatrick, Jim 69

L

laxative abuse 34, 108–112. *See
also* bulimia; drug abuse; purging
Leibel, Rudolph 81–82, 140

M

magazines, teen 117–118
magic-food diets 91–92
Maine, Margo 93
major depression 43
males, eating disorders in. *See* eating
disorders in men and boys
manic episodes 43
mannequins 116
meal-replacement diets 93
media and eating disorders 112–
121. *See also* advertising; eating
disorders, causes of; Internet; peer
pressure
advertising 94–95, 116–117
bigorexia and 22, 73
body types and artistic techniques
119
comparison of American females to
TV counterparts 113, 114
fad diets and 94–96
influence of 58–59, 155
Internet. *See* Internet
models and mannequins 116

music 115
studies on 112–114
subliminal messages in 119
television/movies 114–115
medications. *See also* diet pills; drug
abuse
antidepressants 18–19, 36, 48, 168
for bulimia 36
laxatives 34, 108–112
for treatment of eating disorders
168–169
MEDLINEplus Health Information
184
Mental Health America 44
Meridia 51
Mexican Americans 79
Mikami, Amori 54
Minnesota Twin Family Study 56
models
compared to average American
woman 58, 59
media and 115–116
Monroe, Marilyn 114
morbidity and mortality 121–125
comorbidity 124
populations most affected 123–124
rates of illness and death 122–123
mortality rates. *See* morbidity and
mortality
muscle dysmorphia. *See* bigorexia
MyPyramid 130–132, 174

N

National Academy of Sciences (NAS)
40
National Association of Anorexia
Nervosa and Associated Disorders
(ANAD) 2, 4, 16
contact information 184–185
on morbidity and mortality rates
121, 123–124
support groups through 169
on women and eating disorders
177

National Comorbidity Survey
Replication 121, 123
National Eating Disorders Association
(NEDA) 2, 121
  on binge-eating disorder 29–30
  on body image 154
  contact information 185
  on ethnicity 76
  GO GIRLS! 147
  on prevention 181
  on women and eating disorders 177
National Health and Nutrition
Examination Survey 136
National Heart, Lung and Blood
Institute (NHLBI) 141
National Institute of Diabtes and
Digestive and Kidney Diseases 28
National Institute of Mental Health
(NIMH)
  anorexia, statistics of 15
  binge-eating disorder 28
  on depression 42, 45
  genetics 80
  Internet 107
  male victims 2, 15
  morbidity and mortality rates 121,
  123
  on purging 150
  suicide 9
National Institute on Drug Abuse
24–25
National Institutes of Health (NIH)
  on anorexia 16
  contact information 185
  diet pills, studies on 52
  mentioned 118–119
National Weight Control Registry 89
Native Americans 77
NEDA. See National Eating Disorders
Association (NEDA)
Nemours Foundation's Center for
Children's Health Media
  on binge-eating disorder 30
  on self-image 156

neurotransmitters 56
New England Journal of Medicine
56, 80, 81–82, 92, 121
NHLBI 141
Nielsen Media Research 114
NIH. See National Institutes of Health
(NIH)
NIMH. See National Institute of
Mental Health (NIMH)
nutritional rehabilitation 36. See also
treatment
nutrition and nutritional deficiencies
125–135. See also caloric intake
and expenditures; fad diets; obesity;
weight control
  balanced diets 130–131
  healthy/unhealthy eating habits
  125–127
  informational sources of 95–96
  mistakes, common 127–128
  serving, defined 133
  teenager nutritional needs 128–
  129
  vegetarian diets 133–134
Nutrition and Your Health: Dietary
Guidelines for Americans 185
Nutrition and You: Trends 2002 95

O

OA 170, 185–186
obesity 135–144. See also body
mass index (BMI); caloric intake and
expenditures; exercise; nutrition
and nutritional deficiencies; weight
control
  assessing 141–142
  body fat 139–140
  genetics and 81–82, 141–142
  health problems associated with
  137–139
  statistics 126, 127, 136
  stress as cause of 159
  teenagers and 142–143
Orbach, Susie 117

outpatient care for eating disorder patients 165
Overeaters Anonymous (OA) 170, 185–186
overeating. *See* eating disorders, causes of; obesity
over-the-counter drugs
 diet pills 51–53
 laxatives 108–109

P
Pediatrics (magazine) 77
peer pressure 42, **145–148**. *See also* eating disorders, causes of; self-image
peer support 147
Pew Internet & American Life Project 103
Pope, Harrison, Jr. 22
pregnancy 30–31
Pritts, Sarah 122, 178
pro-ana/pro-mia Web sites 145, 180
Psychological Medicine 19
Psychology of Women Quarterly 78, 180
Psychology Today 160
Psychosomatic Medicine 124
psychotherapy 18, 19, 36, 165–166
purging 2, **149–153**. *See also* bulimia

Q
questions and answers
 anorexia 15, 18, 19
 bigorexia 23
 binge-eating disorder 29, 30
 bulimia 32, 34–35, 35–36
 caloric intake and expenditures 40
 depression and weight 45–46, 48
 eating disorders, causes of 61
 eating disorders, symptoms and diagnosis of 63, 70
 ethnicity and genetics 77
 exercise 88, 90

fad diets 92–93
food allergies 99–100, 101
laxative abuse 109–110
media and eating disorders 117–118, 118–119
nutrition and nutritional deficiencies 133
obesity 140–141
stress and eating habits 159, 162
treatment 166–167, 169
weight control 175–176
women and eating disorders 180

R
Rader Programs 186
RAND Corporation 52
The Real Truth About Beauty 117
recovery. *See* treatment
rehabilitation. *See* treatment
relapses, risk of
 bulimia and 36, 151
 health care professionals and 164
 statistics of 10, 19
Rembrandt Van Rijn 119
Renfrew Center 186
Renoir, Pierre Auguste 119
Rethinking Schools Online 116
reverse anorexia. *See* bigorexia
risk factors 3, 78–79. *See also* eating disorders, causes of
risky business self-test 10–12
Rubens, Peter Paul 119

S
Sacker, Ira 71
SADD 147
Satcher, David 138
schools, involvement in treating eating disorders 172
secretive behavior 5, 29, 109
selective serotonin reuptake inhibitors (SSRIs) 168
self-esteem. *See also* self-image
 body image and 5–6
 peer pressure and 145

self-image. *See* self-image
  stress and 159
self-image **153–158**. *See also* self-
esteem
  body image and 5–6
  eating disorders, symptoms and
    diagnosis of and 69–70
sex abuse 69
Smolak, Linda 58
social interaction
  disrupted by eating disorders 8–9,
    55, 66
  treatment and 171–172
social networks 107
Something Fishy 186
South Beach Diet 92
Spears, Britney 113
SSRIs 168
Stanford University, Internet usage
  study by 106
steroids 24–25
stress and eating habits **158–163**
Striegel-Moore, Ruth H. 76
Students Against Drunk Driving
  (SADD) 147
Stunkard, Albert 80, 81, 82
subliminal messages 119
suicide 9–10, 15, 44, 122
support groups 18, 169–170
Surgeon General's Office 40
Susman, Jeffrey 122, 178

T

teenagers, eating habits of 3
teens speak
  anorexia 19–20
  binge-eating disorder 26–27
  bulimia 36–37
  depression 46–47
  eating disorders, symptoms and
    diagnosis of 66–67
  exercise 86–87
  fad diets 97–98
  males and eating disorders
    74–75

media and eating disorders 119–
  120
nutrition and nutritional
  deficiencies 134–135
obesity 143–144
purging 151–152
self-image 156–158
support groups 170–171
television. *See* media and eating
  disorders
tests
  phsychological 7–8
  self-test 10–12
therapy. *See specific types of therapy*;
  treatment
Time (magazine) 104
treatment **163–173**. *See also*
  medications
  about 8
  behavior modification 166–167,
    172–173
  effectiveness of 10, *171*
  forms of 164–167
  medications. *See* medications
  support groups 169–170
twin studies 80–81

U

U.S. Department of Agriculture
  (USDA)
  caloric intake and 39–40
  on exercise 83–84
  guidelines of 92, 141
  MyPyramid 174
  nutrition and nutritional
    deficiencies 125–126, 130
U.S. Department of Health and
  Human Services (DHHS) 83, 125–
  126, 139, 174
U.S. News and World Report 129

V

vegan diets 133
vegetarian diets 133–134
vomiting. *See* purging

W

WebMD 186
weight and social acceptance. *See* ethnicity and eating disorders; peer pressure; self-image
weight control **174–177**. *See also* caloric intake and expenditures; diet pills; nutrition and nutritional deficiencies; obesity
  about 174–175
  becoming too thin 17–18
  binge-eating disorder and 26
  developing lifelong habits and 177
  students attempting *142*
  unintentional weight loss 176–177
Weight-control Information Network 30, 31
Wing, Rena 89
women and eating disorders **177–181**. *See also* eating disorders in men and boys
  causes 179
  males, females compared 179–180
  prevention 181
  statistics 178
Woodside, D. Blake 72

X

Xenical 50–51

Y

Yale's Center for Eating and Weight Disorders 117
YM (magazine) 117–118
Youth Risk Behavior Surveillance study (2007) 42–43, *44*
Youth Risk Behavior Surveillance System 71, 187
Youth Risk Behavior Survey 3, 33, 84, 127, 142–143
yo-yo dieting. *See* fad diets